Cases on Teaching Pharmacology to Complementary and Alternative Medicine Students

Muhammad Shahzad Aslam
School of Traditional Chinese Medicine, Xiamen University Malaysia, Malaysia

A volume in the Advances in Medical Education, Research, and Ethics (AMERE) Book Series

IGI Global
PUBLISHER of TIMELY KNOWLEDGE

Published in the United States of America by
IGI Global
Medical Information Science Reference (an imprint of IGI Global)
701 E. Chocolate Avenue
Hershey PA, USA 17033
Tel: 717-533-8845
Fax: 717-533-8661
E-mail: cust@igi-global.com
Web site: http://www.igi-global.com

Library of Congress Cataloging-in-Publication Data

Names: Aslam, Muhammad Shahzad, 1985- editor.
Title: Cases on teaching pharmacology to complementary and alternative medicine students / edited by Muhammad Shahzad Aslam.
Description: Hershey, PA : Medical Information Science Reference, [2023] | Includes bibliographical references and index. | Summary: "This book will aim to provide relevant knowledge and skills for an effective teaching pharmacology. It will be written for academician and students who want to improve their understanding drug classification, drug-herb adverse effect, pharmacokinetics and pharmacodynamic of alternative medicine, clinical pharmacology and the use of medical art in teaching pharmacology"-- Provided by publisher.
Identifiers: LCCN 2022061564 (print) | LCCN 2022061565 (ebook) | ISBN 9781668478288 (hardcover) | ISBN 9781668478295 (ebook)
Subjects: MESH: Pharmacology--education | Complementary Therapies--education | Drug Interactions
Classification: LCC RM300 (print) | LCC RM300 (ebook) | NLM QV 18 | DDC 615.1071--dc23/eng/20230221
LC record available at https://lccn.loc.gov/2022061564
LC ebook record available at https://lccn.loc.gov/2022061565

This book is published in the IGI Global book series Advances in Medical Education, Research, and Ethics (AMERE) (ISSN: 2475-6601; eISSN: 2475-661X)

British Cataloguing in Publication Data
A Cataloguing in Publication record for this book is available from the British Library.
All work contributed to this book is new, previously-unpublished material.
The views expressed in this book are those of the authors, but not necessarily of the publisher.
For electronic access to this publication, please contact: eresources@igi-global.com.

Advances in Medical Education, Research, and Ethics (AMERE) Book Series

ISSN:2475-6601
EISSN:2475-661X

MISSION

Humans are living longer now than ever as a result of advances in the medical field. Having the tools available to train knowledgeable and ethical future generations of doctors and medical researchers is essential to continuing to advance our understanding of the human body and develop new ways of treating and curing sickness and disease.

The **Advances in Medical Education, Research, and Ethics (AMERE)** book series highlights publications pertaining to advancements in pedagogical practice for developing future healthcare professionals, research methods, and advancements in the medical field, as well as moral behavior and practice of healthcare professionals, students, and researchers. Featuring research-based book publications that are highly relevant to the healthcare community, this series is ideally designed for library inclusion at medical universities and research institutions as well as personal use by medical professionals, researchers, and upper-level students entering the field.

COVERAGE

- Clinical Research
- Conflicts of Interest
- Ethics in Medicine
- Healthcare Pedagogy
- Medical Curricula
- Medical Simulation
- Patient Data
- Professional Development
- Research Methods
- Scientific Misconduct

IGI Global is currently accepting manuscripts for publication within this series. To submit a proposal for a volume in this series, please contact our Acquisition Editors at Acquisitions@igi-global.com or visit: http://www.igi-global.com/publish/.

The Advances in Medical Education, Research, and Ethics (AMERE) Book Series (ISSN 2475-6601) is published by IGI Global, 701 E. Chocolate Avenue, Hershey, PA 17033-1240, USA, www.igi-global.com. This series is composed of titles available for purchase individually; each title is edited to be contextually exclusive from any other title within the series. For pricing and ordering information please visit http://www.igi-global.com/book-series/advances-medical-education-research-ethics/132365. Postmaster: Send all address changes to above address.

Titles in this Series

For a list of additional titles in this series, please visit:
http://www.igi-global.com/book-series/advances-medical-education-research-ethics/132365

Cases on Diversity, Equity, and Inclusion for the Health Professions Educator
Chasity Beth O'Malley (Wright State University Boonshoft School of Medicine, USA) Arkene Levy (Nova Southeastern University Dr. Kiran C. Patel College of Allopathic Medicine, USA) Amanda Chase (Nova Southeastern University Dr. Kiran C. Patel College of Allopathic Medicine, USA) and Samiksha Prasad (Nova Southeastern University Dr. Kiran C. Patel College of Allopathic Medicne, USA)
Medical Information Science Reference • © 2023 • 369pp • H/C (ISBN: 9781668454930) • US $295.00

Contemporary Issues in Global Medicine and Moving Toward International Healthcare Equity
Nick Comninellis (University of Missouri-Kansas City, USA) and Steven D. Waldman (University of Missouri-Kansas City School of Medicne, USA)
Medical Information Science Reference • © 2022 • 463pp • H/C (ISBN: 9781799884903) • US $325.00

Simulation and Game-Based Learning for the Health Professions
Rachel Umoren (University of Washington, USA)
Medical Information Science Reference • © 2022 • 275pp • H/C (ISBN: 9781799843788) • US $270.00

Handbook of Research on Developing Competencies for Pre-Health Professional Students, Advisors, and Programs
Rohini Ganjoo (The George Washington University, USA) and Lisa S. Schwartz (The George Washington University, USA)
Medical Information Science Reference • © 2022 • 492pp • H/C (ISBN: 9781668459690) • US $470.00

For an entire list of titles in this series, please visit:
http://www.igi-global.com/book-series/advances-medical-education-research-ethics/132365

IGI Global
PUBLISHER of TIMELY KNOWLEDGE

701 East Chocolate Avenue, Hershey, PA 17033, USA
Tel: 717-533-8845 x100 • Fax: 717-533-8661
E-Mail: cust@igi-global.com • www.igi-global.com

Editorial Advisory Board

Wang Yinuo, *School of Traditional Chinese Medicine, Xiamen University Malaysia, Malaysia*
Muhammad Nasir Younis, *Shifa Clinical Research Center, Shifa International Hospital, Islamabad, Pakistan*

Table of Contents

Foreword xvii

Preface xix

Acknowledgment xxii

Chapter 1
Teaching Drug Interactions to Complementary and Alternative Medicine Students: Why Teach Drug Interactions in Complementary and Alternative Medicine? 1
Thaw Zin, Universiti Tunku Abdul Rahman, Malaysia

Chapter 2
Food-Drug Interactions: Types, Causal Mechanisms, Potential Consequences, and Preventive Strategies 21
Muhammad Adil, University of Veterinary and Animal Sciences Lahore, Jhang, Pakistan & Jhang Campus, Pakistan
Muhammad Asif, DHQ Teaching Hospital, Mardan, Pakistan

Chapter 3
A Study of Third-Semester Traditional Chinese Medicine Science Students 38
Yinuo Wang, Xiamen University Malaysia, Malaysia

Chapter 4
A Bio-Therapeutically Squalene: Case Review for T&CM Students as a Wound-Healing Compound 53
Muhammad Shahzad Aslam, School of Traditional Chinese Medicine, Xiamen University Malaysia, Malaysia
Yun Jin Kim, School of Traditional Chinese Medicine, Xiamen University Malaysia, Malaysia
Qian Linchao, School of Traditional Chinese Medicine, Xiamen University Malaysia, Malaysia

Chapter 5
Educating Pharmacology to T&CM Students Using Mnemonics 66
Muhammad Shahzad Aslam, School of Traditional Chinese Medicine, Xiamen University Malaysia, Malaysia

Chapter 6
Enhancing Memory Using Mnemonics Acronym: An Undergraduate Traditional Chinese Medicine Pharmacology Course 73
Muhammad Shahzad Aslam, School of Traditional Chinese Medicine, Xiamen University Malaysia, Malaysia
Dulmaa Lkhagvasuren, Independent Researcher, Mongolia

Chapter 7
Study on the Application of Music Memory Method in Pharmacology 104
Yusu Wang, Xiamen University, China

Chapter 8
Teaching Pharmacology to Complementary and Alternative Medicine Students 116
Muhammad Asif, The Islamia University of Bahawalpur, Pakistan
Rabia Zahid, The Islamia University of Bahawalpur, Pakistan
Misbah Firdous, The Islamia University of Bahawalpur, Pakistan
Ahsan Zahid, The Islamia University of Bahawalpur, Pakistan
Uzma Bashir, The Islamia University of Bahawalpur, Pakistan
Muhammad Hasnain, The Islamia University of Bahawalpur, Pakistan

Chapter 9
Pharmacological Evidence on Drug-Herbal Interactions on the Human Body: Drug-herb Interactions Between Cardiovascular Drugs and Chinese Herbs 130
Tan Chia Hui, Xiamen University Malaysia, Malaysia
Jian Xin Chu, Xiamen University Malaysia, Malaysia
Wen Wen Lee, Xiamen University Malaysia, Malaysia
Ching Hua Ng, Xiamen University Malaysia, Malaysia

Chapter 10
What Pharmacological Evidence Exists for Drug-Herbal Interactions on the Human Body? 141
Joycelyn Chai, Xiamen University Malaysia, Malaysia
Shu Min Chow, Xiamen University Malaysia, Malaysia
Hou Yee Wong, Xiamen University Malaysia, Malaysia
Sock Yan Yap, Xiamen University Malaysia, Malaysia

Chapter 11
A Field Study for Milk Safety and Quality Determination of Heavy Metal Concentration in Raw Milk: Dairy Science ad Technology 150
Bardhyl Limani, Faculty of Food Technology and Nutrition, University of Tetovo, North Macedonia
Mohammad Ayaz Ahmad, University of Guyana, Guyana
Vesna Karapetkovska Hristova, University of St. Kliment Ohridski, Bitola, North Macedonia
Antalov Jagnandan, University of Guyana, Guyana
Syed Khalid Mustafa, University of Tabuk, Saudi Arabia
Jalal Hasan Baker, University of Tabuk, Saudi Arabia
Samira Jebahi, National Center for Sciences and Nuclear Technologies, BiotechPole, Tunisia
Mohammad Rehan Ajmal, University of Tabuk, Saudi Arabia
Abdul Mosawir Quraishi, Qassim University, Saudi Arabia

Compilation of References 183

About the Contributors 205

Index 208

Detailed Table of Contents

Foreword xvii

Preface xix

Acknowledgment xxii

Chapter 1
Teaching Drug Interactions to Complementary and Alternative Medicine Students: Why Teach Drug Interactions in Complementary and Alternative Medicine? 1
Thaw Zin, Universiti Tunku Abdul Rahman, Malaysia

A drug interaction occurs when a patient's response to a drug is modified by food, nutritional supplements, formulation excipients, environmental factors, other drugs, or disease. An interaction can either increase or decrease the effectiveness and/or the side effects of a drug, or it can create a new side effect not seen before. Interactions between drugs (drug-drug interactions) are the commonest and may be either beneficial or harmful. Drug interactions are avoidable and knowing how drug interactions occur, recognizing them when they occur, and knowing how to manage them is an important part of clinical practice. The main objective of learning pharmacology and drug interactions by the CAM students is the integration between the two systems of medicine and as far as the use of medicines are concerned, knowledge of pharmacology and its basic principles are most essential in understanding the adverse reactions and drug interactions that can hamper the integrating of the two systems of medicine as such outcomes will produce doubts and lack of confidence in the end-users.

Chapter 2
Food-Drug Interactions: Types, Causal Mechanisms, Potential Consequences, and Preventive Strategies 21
Muhammad Adil, University of Veterinary and Animal Sciences Lahore, Jhang, Pakistan & Jhang Campus, Pakistan
Muhammad Asif, DHQ Teaching Hospital, Mardan, Pakistan

Bioactive dietary ingredients can influence the pharmacokinetic and/or pharmacodynamic attributes of drugs that are orally administered either in conjunction with food or following a short interval. The pharmacokinetic form of food-drug interactions is reflected by changes in the rate/extent of drug absorption, distribution, metabolism, or excretion. Whereas, diet-induced pharmacodynamic modulation may arise in terms of additive, synergistic, or antagonistic effects. Most of the clinically important, food-drug interactions occur on account of altered drug bioavailability attributed to dietary constituents. Depending upon their occurrence and severity, food-drug interactions leading to enhanced plasma drug concentrations may have beneficial or harmful consequences. The outcomes of food-drug interactions may range from the loss of drug efficacy and subsequent treatment failure to serious adverse effects. Proper adherence to the drug-specific prescribing guidelines and patient compliance are requisite for minimizing the likelihood of potential food-drug interactions.

Chapter 3
A Study of Third-Semester Traditional Chinese Medicine Science Students 38
Yinuo Wang, Xiamen University Malaysia, Malaysia

Pharmacology is an important and compulsory subject for undergraduate traditional Chinese medicine (TCM) science students. However, at this stage, the third semester TCM science students still have some misunderstanding and neglects about pharmacology. The research method was conducted by interviewing four undergraduate TCM science students who had graduated and were planning to gain their next degree in different fields in terms of pharmacology studies methods, application of pharmacology knowledge, and perceptions of pharmacology. The study found third semester undergraduate TCM science students had difficulties in learning pharmacology. However, the use of mnemonics, scenario simulation, literature writing and reading, etc. helped to motivate students and assisted in memorizing relevant knowledge points. Third semester TCM science students should pay attention to the study of pharmacology and find appropriate method in the meantime. In addition, educators and educational institutions are recommended to adjust teaching strategies according to students' status.

Chapter 4
A Bio-Therapeutically Squalene: Case Review for T&CM Students as a Wound-Healing Compound 53
Muhammad Shahzad Aslam, School of Traditional Chinese Medicine, Xiamen University Malaysia, Malaysia
Yun Jin Kim, School of Traditional Chinese Medicine, Xiamen University Malaysia, Malaysia
Qian Linchao, School of Traditional Chinese Medicine, Xiamen University Malaysia, Malaysia

Although the skin tissue on our bodies is a well-organized structure with high biomechanical properties like tensile strength and friction, we have all experienced various types of wounds throughout our lives owing to numerous etiological factors. In the general population, it is a substantial source of morbidity. For instance, in the case of burnt skin tissue, self-healing is in fact a large and challenging barrier to tissue regeneration. Squalene is a bioactive triterpene that occurs naturally and plays a key role in the process of making sterols. The most well-known source of squalene is shark liver oil. Vegetable oils may contain squalene in a range of concentrations. They have been extracted using a variety of techniques, including supercritical carbon dioxide, microwave, ultrasonic, cold press, and traditional Soxhlet extractions. In vitro and in animal models, these substances have been demonstrated to have anticancer, antioxidant, drug carrier, detoxifier, skin moisturising, and emollient effects.

Chapter 5
Educating Pharmacology to T&CM Students Using Mnemonics 66
Muhammad Shahzad Aslam, School of Traditional Chinese Medicine, Xiamen University Malaysia, Malaysia

The scientific field of pharmacology aims to give a thorough understanding of how medications affect the human body. In Malaysia, the bachelor's degree programme of traditional Malay medicine, traditional Chinese medicine, acupuncture, Moxibustion and Tuina, Siddha medicine, homeopathy, chiropractic, and osteopathy contain two credit hours for the subject pharmacology. The student faces a time challenge to understand the broad concept of pharmacology and memorising some important drugs classification. Therefore, using mnemonic is an interesting method to develop and understanding and memorising drug classifications.

Chapter 6
Enhancing Memory Using Mnemonics Acronym: An Undergraduate Traditional Chinese Medicine Pharmacology Course 73
Muhammad Shahzad Aslam, School of Traditional Chinese Medicine, Xiamen University Malaysia, Malaysia
Dulmaa Lkhagvasuren, Independent Researcher, Mongolia

Traditional Chinese medicine students find pharmacology challenging because it is complicated, yet they still need to understand facts about the mechanism of actions of drugs and how to use this knowledge in clinical settings. Mnemonics are strategies that can enhance learning and memory of course material. Mnemonics are memory techniques that aid in chunking and organising material to be learnt; as a result, they improve encoding and ease retrieval. There are variety of forms that include acronyms and acrostics (also known as first-letter mnemonics), the loci method, the pegword method, the keyword approach, auditory, visual, and kinesthetic mnemonics, and a group of semantic-based mnemonic devices such as rhymes, songs, and stories.

Chapter 7
Study on the Application of Music Memory Method in Pharmacology 104
Yusu Wang, Xiamen University, China

Memory is the faculty by which the mind stores and remembers information. Music is some combination of vocal or instrumental sounds. Research offers new insights into how music links to memories, and how those connections make life better. Medicine is undoubtedly one of the most challenging courses for memory. In all academic settings, there is no other need for powerful mnemonic tools like medicine. In the study of pharmacology, students generally report that the course of pharmacology is difficult, some students say that the names of drugs are too complicated to remember; however, few students realize that music mnemonics is a good way to learn.

Chapter 8
Teaching Pharmacology to Complementary and Alternative Medicine Students....................116
Muhammad Asif, The Islamia University of Bahawalpur, Pakistan
Rabia Zahid, The Islamia University of Bahawalpur, Pakistan
Misbah Firdous, The Islamia University of Bahawalpur, Pakistan
Ahsan Zahid, The Islamia University of Bahawalpur, Pakistan
Uzma Bashir, The Islamia University of Bahawalpur, Pakistan
Muhammad Hasnain, The Islamia University of Bahawalpur, Pakistan

The field of complementary medicine (CM) is still thriving in several nations. A rise in enrollment at CM educational establishments in both public and private tertiary sectors has indeed been tightly linked to the global popularity of CM. This work presents the very first critical analysis of relevant research analyzing CM education research in direct response to this significant gap. 18 publications out of the 9496 that were found matched the study's criteria for inclusion (English language, kind of CM professionals' education), and they focused on four main problems: CM educational offerings and provision; the development of educational competencies to develop clinical skills and standards; the application of new educational theory, methods and technology in CM; and future challenges facing CM education. This critical integrative review highlights two key issues of interest and significance for CM educational institutions, CM regulators, and researchers, and points to a number of significant gaps in this area of research.

Chapter 9
Pharmacological Evidence on Drug-Herbal Interactions on the Human Body: Drug-herb Interactions Between Cardiovascular Drugs and Chinese Herbs.....130
Tan Chia Hui, Xiamen University Malaysia, Malaysia
Jian Xin Chu, Xiamen University Malaysia, Malaysia
Wen Wen Lee, Xiamen University Malaysia, Malaysia
Ching Hua Ng, Xiamen University Malaysia, Malaysia

Assessing the potential herb-drug interactions is necessary to ensure clinical safety and to prevent any untoward effects. Studies have identified a variety of adverse effects on herb-drug interactions. Common mechanisms include the modulation of drug-metabolic enzymes, which leads to irreversible impacts. Physicians should constantly double-check if patients see numerous prescribers or visit multiple hospital settings before prescribing drugs to avoid pharmaceutical toxicity. Chinese herbal medicines are an essential part of TCM practice. Thus, the elevation and classification of toxic herb-drug interactions are helpful to ensure the safet usage by practitioners in optimizing the effectiveness of treatment strategies. According to

WHO, cardiovascular diseases caused about 17.9 million deaths, accounting for 32% of all global deaths in 2019. This literature review will be focusing on cardiovascular drugs due to the high global mortality rate of cardiovascular diseases.

Chapter 10
What Pharmacological Evidence Exists for Drug-Herbal Interactions on the Human Body? 141
Joycelyn Chai, Xiamen University Malaysia, Malaysia
Shu Min Chow, Xiamen University Malaysia, Malaysia
Hou Yee Wong, Xiamen University Malaysia, Malaysia
Sock Yan Yap, Xiamen University Malaysia, Malaysia

Chinese herbal medicine is one of the treatment pathways amongst the multicomponent therapeutics of traditional Chinese medicine (TCM). The main role of it includes regaining homeostasis, stabilizing health, preventing illnesses, and overall, prolonging life span and improving quality of life. Since TCM is more focused on treating the root of diseases, Chinese herbal medicine can also be used to prevent, treat, and manage various chronic diseases, such as cardiovascular diseases, musculoskeletal disorders, neurological disorders, and so on. Other significant roles can also be seen as to alleviate several side effects of Western medicine's treatment and be incorporated as part of the management process of the disease recovery and rehabilitation period.

Chapter 11
A Field Study for Milk Safety and Quality Determination of Heavy Metal Concentration in Raw Milk: Dairy Science ad Technology 150
Bardhyl Limani, Faculty of Food Technology and Nutrition, University of Tetovo, North Macedonia
Mohammad Ayaz Ahmad, University of Guyana, Guyana
Vesna Karapetkovska Hristova, University of St. Kliment Ohridski, Bitola, North Macedonia
Antalov Jagnandan, University of Guyana, Guyana
Syed Khalid Mustafa, University of Tabuk, Saudi Arabia
Jalal Hasan Baker, University of Tabuk, Saudi Arabia
Samira Jebahi, National Center for Sciences and Nuclear Technologies, BiotechPole, Tunisia
Mohammad Rehan Ajmal, University of Tabuk, Saudi Arabia
Abdul Mosawir Quraishi, Qassim University, Saudi Arabia

In this chapter, a modest attempt has been made to study the heavy metal contamination including their bio-accumulation and toxic effects in our daily lives. It is the alarming hazards to the environment, especially in the industrial zones, that confirm the attention paid to these contaminants. The authors tried to determine the content of heavy metals (cadmium - Cd, lead - Pb, copper - Cu, zinc - Zn, nickel - Ni, manganese – Mn, and chromium - Cr) in the individual samples of cow milk from the farms in seven different localities. The distribution and dynamics of the determined heavy metals in the milk were recorded at different distances starting from the area of the industrial capacity. All the milk samples were analyzed properly, and the authors did chemical consumption and somatic cells and bacteria inside them. The findings were found within good agreements with others.

Compilation of References 183

About the Contributors 205

Index 208

Foreword

Cases on Teaching Pharmacology to Complementary and Alternative Medicine Students has emphasised the importance of the subject pharmacology to traditional and complementary medicine students (T&CM). The first chapter has focused on teaching drug interactions to T&CM students. The author has focused that health care professionals should minimize the risks of drug interactions by an accurate management such as dose adjustment, spacing of dosing times, and close monitoring of therapy in drug combinations. If dosage adjustment is ineffective, the drug should be replaced by one that does not interact with other drugs being taken. The next chapter has explained the importance of the merging field of nutrigenomics that can be applied to explore the interface between dietary substances and genomic factors for explicating the cellular and molecular basis of food-drug interactions. The third authors have discussed the methodology of pharmacology study for undergraduate Traditional Chinese medicine students. The author found out that traditional Chinese medicine undergraduates are generally not good at memorizing and mastering pharmacology courses, which is related to the different theoretical systems of Chinese and western medicine. Dr. Muhammad Shahzad Aslam and his co researcher have focused in next chapter about the bioactive metabolites in medicinal plants such as squalene as a natural wound healing compound. Moreover, in fifth and sixth chapter, the authors have written a book chapter to give the method to memorize the easiest way to study drugs by using the suffix in a drug name. Traditional Chinese medicine students find pharmacology challenging because it is complicated, yet they still need to understand facts about the mechanism of actions of drugs and how to use this knowledge in clinical settings. The authors have suggested to used Mnemonic to memorize it quickly. The next chapter (Chapter 7) written by Yusu wang has given a new direction of enhancing memory of mind using music to memorize drug information. Chapter 8 briefly explain to audience in maintaining the ethical and efficient therapeutic interventions using complementary medicine (CM), that is required in the continuous creation of minimal professional standards. The author has focused to developed CM as highly competent and educated health system in the future and proposed integration of valuable conventional homeopathic concepts, together with the establishment of suitable regulatory mechanisms. Chapter 9 will consist of the literature review that focused on reported Drug-herb interactions between cardiovascular drugs and Chinese herbs. Chapter 10 has raised some safety issues related to Chinese herbal medicines. The authors have discussed with few examples regarding drug-herb interactions in context to Cytochrome P450 3A4. The last chapter has discussed about a field Study for milk safety and quality. The study has determined the heavy metal concentration in raw milk in the Polog region.

Kapil Kumar
Uttarakhand Technical University, India

Preface

Traditional and complementary medicine (T&CM) has gained attention during the past ten years. T&CM has been widely used by people all around the world for many years. Complementary and alternative medicine use in the middle east was valued at USD 8,176.4 million in 2022 and is expected to expand at a compound annual growth rate (CAGR) of 20.18% from 2023 to 2030. Up to 80% of the population in Pakistan use CAM, including herbal products, in their daily practice (Shaikh et al., 2009). Traditional Chinese Medicine (TCM) is a cultural treasure that has been preserved by Chinese civilization for more than 5000 years. It has a wide range of therapeutic uses and has developed a distinctive theoretical framework that is crucial to the country's health (Guo et al, 2022).

T&CM has been categorized into traditional Malay medicine, traditional Chinese medicine, traditional Indian medicine, homeopathy, chiropractic, osteopathy, and Islamic medical practice (According to the ministry of health Malaysia). There seems to be a 'problem' for T&CM students in understanding western medicine subjects. Pharmacology is one of the basic medical science subjects. It combines information from a variety of scientific fields, such as chemistry, biochemistry, molecular biology, and physiology, and has a major beneficial effect on human health. Numerous medical therapies are built on the scientific understanding developed from pharmacologic investigations.

THE CHALLENGES

- The challenge of establishing a good understanding of the drug mechanism of action among T&CM students.
- The challenge in understanding drug-herbal interactions and drug-food interactions. Medicinal herbs are complex of several bioactive compounds and students need to develop rationality in their treatment and management of the disease.

- The challenge of establishing a balanced treatment of western and eastern medicine. T&CM students need to understand the importance of pharmacology as one of the important pillars of western medicine.

The development of different teaching pedagogies has been discussed in a different book chapter. Moreover, the current book emphasizes the importance of pharmacology as a subject and gives directions to different learning strategies. About 25% of the prescriptions worldwide are filled with drugs that are obtained or extracted from plant sources (Tyler et al., 1998). Therefore, T&CM students must learn and understand the pharmacology of drugs, mechanism of action, clinical indication, adverse drug reactions, drug interactions, drug-herb interactions, drug nutrition interactions, and contraindications.

ORGANIZATION OF THE BOOK

The book is organized into 11 chapters. A brief description of each of the chapters follows:

Chapter 1 explores teaching drug interactions to complementary and alternative medicine students.

Chapter 2 discusses the food-drug interactions: types, causal mechanisms, potential consequences, and preventive strategies.

Chapter 3 discusses the promotion of different learning methods for pharmacology learning, the appropriate teaching strategies, and the significance of pharmacology for the future development of traditional Chinese medicine students.

Chapter 4 recalls the importance of a bio-therapeutically bioactive squalene in natural medicine as a case review for T&CM students as a wound healing compound. The current case will remind the T&CM students to connect nature with chemistry.

Mnemonic techniques can include songs, poems, rhymes, outlines, images, and acronyms. Mnemonics give meaning to something ordinary to make it more memorable when you try to recall it. Chapter 5 will educate students to study pharmacology using mnemonics.

Chapter 6 explores how traditional Chinese medicine students find pharmacology challenging because it is complicated, yet they still need to understand facts about the mechanism of actions of drugs and how to use this knowledge in clinical settings. Mnemonics are strategies that can enhance learning and memory of course material.

Music is the soul of the universe, but how could music help in studying pharmacology? Chapter 7 discusses the application of the music memory method in Pharmacology.

The increase of complementary medicine (CM) as a subject is increased and to date, no critical analysis of peer-reviewed studies assessing CM academic achievement has been performed. Chapter 8 presents the very first critical analysis of relevant research analyzing CM education research in direct response to this significant gap.

Chapter 9 discusses the literature review that focussed on reported drug-herb interactions between cardiovascular drugs and Chinese herbs.

Chapter 10 has focused on the safety concerns related to Chinese herbal medicines that activate Cytochrome P450 3A4.

Chapter 11 discusses the heavy metal contamination in milk, their bioaccumulation and toxic effects on wildlife.

Muhammad Shahzad Aslam
Xiamen University Malaysia, Malaysia

REFERENCES

Guo, J., Xuan, Z. Y., & Xie, Y. (2020). Problems and considerations in pharmaceutical researches of new traditional Chinese medicine. *Chinese Traditional and Herbal Drugs*, *51*(8), 2267–2272.

Middle East Complementary and Alternative Medicine Market Size, Share, & Trends Analysis Report By Intervention (Traditional Alternative Medicine & Botanicals), By Application, By Distribution Channel, And Segment Forecasts, 2023 – 2030. (n.d.). https://www.grandviewresearch.com/industry-analysis/middle-east-integrative-health-complementary-alternative-medicine-market

Shaikh, S. H., Malik, F., James, H., & Abdul, H. (2009). Trends in the use of complementary and alternative medicine in Pakistan: A population-based survey. *Journal of Alternative and Complementary Medicine*, *15*(5), 545–550. doi:10.1089/acm.2008.0232 PMID:19422284

Tyler, V. E., Brady, L. R., & Robbers, J. E. (1998). *Pharmacognosy* (9th ed.). Lea & Febiger.

Acknowledgment

This book is the product of my teaching career in Malaysia that began around five years ago in Xiamen University Malaysia. Its growth and improvement have been assisted in some manner by several people. I want to thank them for their help, so please accept my gratitude. To start, I would like to extend my sincere gratitude to my advisers Professor Dr Muhammad Syarhabil Ahmad, and Professor Dr. Awang Soh Mamat for their constant encouragement, and support. I want to thanks Professor Dr. Yun Jin Kim and Professor Dr. Qian Linchao for their valuable suggestions and time.

I want to appreciate my all students whom I teach during this journey in Xiamen University Malaysia. I am most grateful for the enthusiasm, active participations of my students during my teaching through which I have taken inspiration to write the book. I am thankful to Wang Yinuo, Yi Lisha, Yu Hanyi, Chong Kar Wai, Wang Yusu, Wang Xinyan, Liying Huang, Tay Si Sheng, Chin Chun Wang whom I had taught as my first batch of traditional Chinese Medicine. A special thanks to Wang Yinuo and Wang Yusu for their active contribution in writing the book chapter which will help the students in future to prepare this subject.I want to appreciate some more students whom suggestions and advice brings me positive energy and motivation to write the book such as Chu Jian Xin, Tan Chia Hui, Tan Celine, Jia Yee Chai, Alanis Tang Kie Yi, Chan Lu Qi, Emily Ng, Joycelyn Chai Le Chin, Ooi Yin Cheah, How Yng Ye, Yap Lay Chin, Chong Jin An, Wong Hou Yee, Poo Rou En, Yap Sock Yan, Chong Jin Wen, Seng Chee Hee, Ann Naomi Wong Hao Wei, Lee Wen Wen, Ng Ching Hua, Tee Niam Chi, Chow Shu Min, Yap Wan Yinn, Koh Shi Lin, Hong Jessie, Fong Jing Ting, How Ye Zhen, Ching Yusheng, and Yee Kai Lee. These are few names of my students whom I still remember in my mind and they give me ideas, feedback in uplifting the subject and motivations to write the book. I apologies from my students if I miss any name as every student is important to me and I appreciate everyone.

I would like to say my thanks to the dean, faculty, and management of school of traditional Chinese Medicine, Xiamen University Malaysia for believing me in my hard work and dedication to write the book for the students who face difficulty in studying pharmacology.

I am thankful to authors (Thaw zin, Wang Yinuo, Wang Yusu, Muhammad Adil, Yun Jin Kim, Qian Linchao, Dulmaa Lkhagvasuren, Muhammad Asif, Rabia Zahid, Misbah Firdous, Ahsan Zahid, Uzma Bashir, Muhammad Hasnain, Joycelyn Chai, Shu Min Chow, Hou Yee Wong, Sock Yan Yap, Bardhyl Limani, Vesna Karapetkovska Hristova, Antalov Jagnandan, M. Ayaz Ahmad, Syed Khalid Mustafa, Jalal. H. Baker, Samira Jebahi, Mohammad Rehan Ajmal, A. M. Quraishi, Chu Jian Xin, Lee Wen Wen, Ng Ching Hua, Tan Chia Hui) for contributing in writing the book.

I appreciate my wife Saima Nisar for providing the necessary support, care and for keeping up the patience during the relatively long process of accomplishing this task.

Chapter 1
Teaching Drug Interactions to Complementary and Alternative Medicine Students:
Why Teach Drug Interactions in Complementary and Alternative Medicine?

Thaw Zin
Universiti Tunku Abdul Rahman, Malaysia

EXECUTIVE SUMMARY

A drug interaction occurs when a patient's response to a drug is modified by food, nutritional supplements, formulation excipients, environmental factors, other drugs, or disease. An interaction can either increase or decrease the effectiveness and/or the side effects of a drug, or it can create a new side effect not seen before. Interactions between drugs (drug-drug interactions) are the commonest and may be either beneficial or harmful. Drug interactions are avoidable and knowing how drug interactions occur, recognizing them when they occur, and knowing how to manage them is an important part of clinical practice. The main objective of learning pharmacology and drug interactions by the CAM students is the integration between the two systems of medicine and as far as the use of medicines are concerned, knowledge of pharmacology and its basic principles are most essential in understanding the adverse reactions and drug interactions that can hamper the integrating of the two systems of medicine as such outcomes will produce doubts and lack of confidence in the end-users.

DOI: 10.4018/978-1-6684-7828-8.ch001

INTRODUCTION

The World Health Organization has estimated that 80% of people worldwide, including highly developed countries, uses herbal medicine and other alternative therapies to maintain health and wellness and to combat illness, especially for minor ailments and chronic co-morbidities (WHO, 2019). Indeed, modern science has made dramatic improvements in medicine and public health where infection, poisoning, injury, nutrition, or personal and environmental hygiene plays a major part in etiology. However, in chronic/degenerative diseases which mainly affects the elderly people, and where other factors such as emotional, behavioral and spiritual factors are involved and interrelated, the results have been less striking, or even disappointing (Gabay & Spencer, 2021; Schmidt-Mende et al., 2019). In addition, scientific view rejects the concept of 'holistic' favoring of treating physical body and mind separately, with specialists even treating body in parts within its domain (Berman, 2001). Modern health and medical services, with their ever-increasing cost, has also been questioned in many quarters (Smith et al., 2009).

Integrating Western and CAM, popularly known as Integrative Medicine, is an approach to medical care that combines conventional medicine with CAM practices that have shown through science to be safe and effective. This approach often stresses the patient's preferences, and it attempts to address the mental, physical, and spiritual aspects of health (Tiralongo & Wallis 2008).

BACKGROUND

Standard medical care is a treatment that is accepted by the medical experts as an evidence-based practice for a certain type of disease, not only taught in Medical Universities but is widely used by healthcare professionals all over the world (Tiralongo & Wallis 2008; Catto et al., 2014). Generally, Allopathic or Western Medicine is currently accepted as the conventional or best practice or standard therapy.

Complementary and alternative medicine (CAM) is the term used for medical products and practices that are not part of Conventional Medicine or standard medical care. Herbal remedies, acupuncture, chiropractic, etc., have continued to grow in popularity and are often referred to many as "natural," "holistic," "home remedy," or "Eastern Medicine". Especially in old age, where it is not just the disease but the interconnectedness of body, mind, and spirit in achieving health and sense of well-being that become the most important factors in life (Kumar-Pal, 2002). As such, it was generally accepted that everyone should have opportunity to access modern technology as well as ancient traditions of healing to be able to live, not just longer but a life that is productive, meaningful and with a purpose (WHO, 2019; Catto et al., 2014).

Western medicine principles are dependent upon scientific research, proven through tests on the body, organs and systems, cellular mechanisms, right down to receptors, signaling pathways, genes, chromosomes and DNA (Brunton et al., 2017; Page et al., 2006). In contrast, principles of CAM rests upon a long history of use; the sum total of the knowledge, skill, and practices based on the theories, beliefs, and experiences indigenous to different cultures, whether explicable or not, has been used in the maintenance of health as well as in the prevention, diagnosis, improvement or treatment of physical and mental illness long before the Western Medicine was known to exist (Kumar-Pal, 2002). Thus, in order to overcome the diversity of principles between the two systems, it is only fair that each will have to have sufficient knowledge of the other in order to reach its goal (Gray et al., 2019). However, as far as the use of medicines are concerned, knowledge of pharmacology and its basic principles are essential, not just for the effective drug therapy in the treatment of diseases, but also in understanding the adverse reactions and drug interactions that can result in the integrating of the two systems of medicine (Brunton et al., 2017; Page et al., 2006). Medicine and many allied medical sciences, have recognized this trend and have integrated their curriculum to acknowledge CAM, and at the same time, it becomes a necessity that students learning CAM accepts and understand that knowledge of pharmacology and its basic principles are essential to make the ends meet, with each complementing each other and removing any implied competition between professionals to achieving the best comprehensive care possible (Catto et al., 2014; Mann et al., 2004).

WESTERN AND TRADITIONAL MEDICINE

The two systems of medicine, Western and Traditional Medicine, are like the two sides of a coin. They cannot be viewed together since the principles and methods are so diverse, yet when used together, they can become a valuable asset reaching the value which individually, can never achieve. Thus, it became a solution that both the system should be integrated and be viewed as collaborators and not competitors and be open to accept the controversies and problems that can come with it including the use of medicines and the reactions and interactions that comes with it (Soliman et al., 2021; Mann et al., 2004). It has been widely accepted that with one system complementing the other, such can offer a way of making the treatment more holistic (Berman, 2001).

Learning Pharmacology by Complementary Alternative Medicine Students

However, the problems relating to integrating the two systems of the medicine, Western and Traditional Medicine, is not just in understanding the diversity of principles, application and use, but also from the likelihood of the combined effects of the medicines used and the interactions that can follow which can be beneficial or deleterious (Christensen et al., 2017; Gray et al., 2019; Snyder et al., 2012) and this should be made aware by all stakeholders concerned, healthcare providers, end-users, their families and the public (Frenkel et al., 2004). Lack of knowledge and awareness is one of the greatest barriers to its appropriate use, with the healthcare providers being unable to provide adequate advice on the safety issues or about the effectiveness of a particular therapy in one end and the conventional care users not sharing the information of its use to the healthcare providers on the other (Thomson et al., 2012; Berman, 2001). As such, many medical schools teaching Western Medicine, now include training programs on complementary and alternative therapies, and curriculum reviews, research and development encouraging the additional skills of openness, sensitivity to cultural influences and beliefs, communication, and critical appraisal of the literature of complementary and alternative therapy treatments have been implemented (Soliman et al., 2021; Berman, 2001; Templeman et al., 2015; Tiralongo & Wallis, 2008). However, the reverse is not true on how western medicine should be integrated and taught to Complementary and Alternative Medicine (CAM) students, which is seriously lacking (Gray et al., 2019; Catto et al., 2014). Review of literature shows numerous studies on how CAM should be taught to medical students, nurses and pharmacists is evident, very little has been done on how pharmacology should be taught to CAM students (Rao et al., 2012). As far as the risks involved in combining the two systems mainly stems from the drug interactions and the rational use of drugs, a considerable challenge exists for the curriculum developers as well as the educators in determining the necessary acquisition of pharmacological knowledge and therapeutics into the CAM curriculum through an evidence-based medicine approach (Soliman et al., 2021; Kennedy, 2019). Since learning drug interactions involves all aspects of basic pharmacology, such as pharmacokinetics, pharmacodynamics and mechanism of drug action, it provides an ideal starting point for instilling the interest and rationale on how and why pharmacology should be learned by the CAM students (Caterina et al., 2013; Page et al., 2006). Since the first pharmacological principle states that it is the 'dose' that decides a poison or a remedy (Brunton, 2017), intelligent planning on the content and mode of delivery of the pharmacology within the CAM curriculum is of utmost importance. One should not lose sight of the objective that learning of pharmacology by the CAM students is the application, the rational use of medicines, and not as to becoming Western

Medicine doctors or pharmacologists (Gray et al., 2019; Catto et al., 2014). The principle is also true in learning drug interactions that common interactions should be the main content, as described in this chapter, not all interactions, but those that can aid in understanding the basic pharmacological principles like pharmacokinetics and altered bioavailability, or pharmacodynamics like potentiation where harmless CAM remedy can increase the toxicity of Western Medicine should be included (Christensen et al., 2017; Committee for Human Medicinal Products, 2012).

THE BASIC PRINCIPLES UNDERLYING DRUG INTERACTIONS

Drug Interactions (Drug-Drug Interactions)

A drug interaction is a reaction between two (or more) drugs or between a drug and a food, beverage, or supplement affecting the activity of a drug, the effects (Moses & McGuire, 2010). The drug whose activity is affected by such interactions is called the object drug, and the agent which precipitates such an interaction is referred to as the precipitant. The resultant effect can be both ways, meaning it can be increased, decreased, or produce new effect that neither produces on its own; may be either desired or undesired, beneficial, or harmful (Snyder et al., 2012). Taking a drug while having certain medical conditions can also cause a drug interaction. Generally, most medications can be safely used with other drugs/medicines, but certain medicines are more prone to cause interactions when used combination and need to be monitored (Brunton et al., 2017).

Figure 1. Object drug interacting with the precipitant to bring about interactions

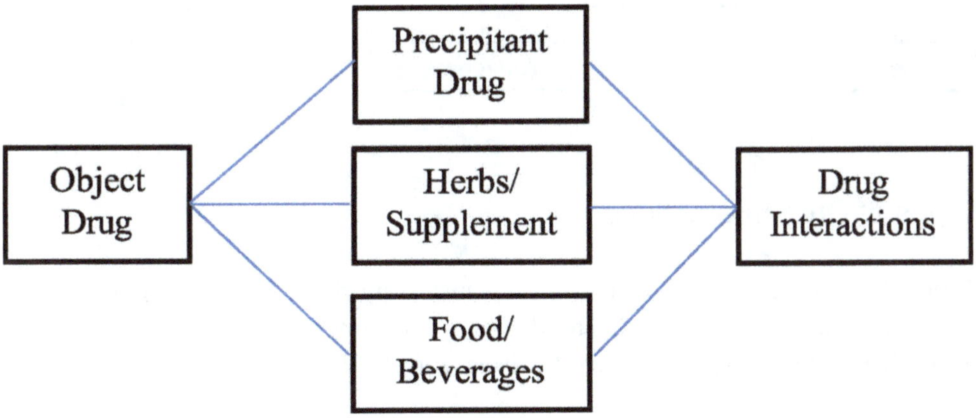

Drug interactions can occur in conditions such as:

- Combining of main drugs with adjuvant (support) drug (as in infection – antibiotics with analgesics)
- Drugs used for current illness with those prescribed for:
  - Chronic diseases – tuberculosis, diabetes, hypertension, psychiatric and heart conditions
  - Prophylactic measures – oral contraceptive pills, oral anticoagulants, depot injection
- Sudden change of one drug to the next before the effect of the former has abated (overlapping/persistence effects)
- Food having active constituents – caffeine, alcohol, cheese

Knowledge of drug interactions enables a physician to minimize or prevent drug toxicity by adjustment of dosage or schedule of drug administration or by choice of an alternative agent (Moses & McGuire, 2010).

Figure 2. Types of drug interactions and the possible consequences

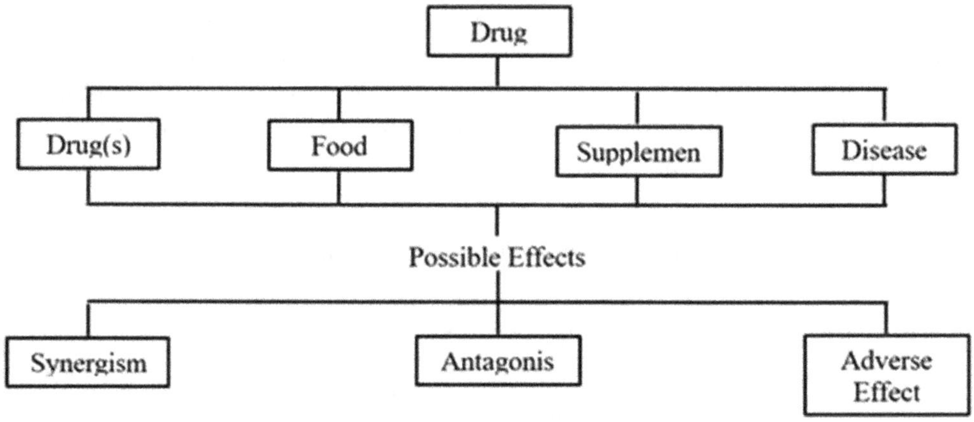

Types of Drug Interactions

Typically, interaction between drugs means (drug-drug interaction). However, interactions may also exist with foods (drug-food interactions), as well as herbs (drug- herb interactions) and even the disease itself (drug-disease).

Mechanisms of Drug Interactions

Interactions between medications (drug-drug interactions) generally fall into one of three main categories:

- **Chemical:** One drug chemical property neutralizing the other.
- **Pharmacokinetics:** Involving absorption, distribution, metabolism, and excretion of one or both of the interacting drugs upon the other.
- **Pharmacodynamics:** Involving the actions of the two interacting drugs.

Pharmacokinetic Drug Interactions

The pharmacological and toxic effects of most therapeutic agents are thought to be related to the concentration of the free drug at the receptor sites which is influenced continuously by the process of absorption, distribution, metabolism, and excretion. If another drug, food, herbs or even the disease itself, can alter the pharmacokinetics of that drug, changes in the duration and intensity of action may result. Such type of drug interactions are referred to as pharmacokinetic drug interactions (Moses & McGuire, 2010; Brunton et al., 2017; Caterina et al., 2013; Snyder et al., 2012).

Absorption

Absorption of drugs from the gastrointestinal tract is dependent on many factors, some of which can be modified by therapeutic agents and may influence the gastrointestinal absorption of other compounds (Caterina et al., 2013). Thus, the gastrointestinal absorption of one drug may be affected by other drugs that bind or chelate or alter the gastrointestinal mobility. Some examples are given in Tables 1 and 2.

Table 1. Some examples of common drug interactions affecting the absorption of drugs into the systemic circulation

Drug-1 (Object)	Drug-2 (Precipitant)	Interaction
Antacids (Ca2+, Mg2+, Al3+), milk	Tetracyclines, ciprofloxacin	Chelation, decrease absorption of drug-2
Ferrous sulphate	Quinolones, thyroid hormones, tetracyclines	Decrease absorption of drug-2
Anticholinergics, antidepressants (having cholinergic effect)	All drugs	Reduced gastric emptying, delay absorption of Drug-2
Metoclopramide	All drugs	Accelerate absorption of Drug-2
Antimicrobials (broad spectrum)	Oral anticoagulent	Potentiate anticoagulant effect
Vasoconstrictors (adrenaline)	Local anesthetics (Lignocain)	Prolong the local anesthetic action

Distribution

Drug interaction can occur during distribution by two mechanisms:

- Displacement from plasma protein binding sites. A drug that is extensively protein-bound can be displaced from its binding sites by a competing drug so raising the free drug concentration of the first drug.
- Displacement from tissue binding sites also tends to increase the blood concentration of the displaced drug (Caterina et al., 2013).

Table 2. Some examples of common drug interactions affecting distribution of drugs within the body

Drug Displaced	Clinical Effects
Sulphonylureas	Enhanced hypoglycemia
Oral anticoagulants	Bleeding
Bilirubin	Kernicterus
Phenytoin	Increased toxicity
Methotrexate/digoxin	Increased effect, increased toxicity

Metabolism

Most drugs are metabolized to inactive/fewer active metabolites by enzymes in liver/intestine. Since only a few different cytochrome P450 isozymes are involved in drug metabolism, competition between two drugs for these isozymes will occasionally occur. The metabolism of drugs can be stimulated or inhibited by concurrent therapy (Snyder et al., 2012).

Prodrugs are drugs that are not active in the form administered to patients and require activation by enzymes in the body before they can produce their effect. Inhibition of the metabolism of these prodrugs may reduce the amount of active drug formed and decrease or eliminate the therapeutic effect.

Drugs, called "enzyme inducers", are capable of increasing the activity of drug metabolizing enzymes, resulting in a decrease in the effect of certain other drugs. These include drugs such as barbiturates, phenytoin, rifampicin, meprobamate, carbamazepine, sulphinpyrazone and griseofulvin (Caterina et al., 2013). Some examples are given in Tables 3 and 4.

Table 3. some examples of common drug interactions resulting from induction of hepatic microsomal enzymes

Drugs Affected	Enzyme Inducer	Effect of Interaction
Oral anticoagulants	Barbiturates, Carbamazepine, Rifampicin	Decreased anticoagulant effect
Oral contraceptives	Barbiturates, Rifampicin, Phenytoin, Carbamazepine	Decreased contraceptive effect, break through bleeding, contraceptive failure
Sulphonylureas	Rifampicin	Decreased hypoglycemic effect
Corticosteroids	Barbiturates, Phenytoin, Carbamazepine	Decreased corticosteroid effects
Phenytoin	Rifampicin	Decreased Phenytion effects, increased seizure risk.
Theophylline	Barbiturates, Rifampicin, Tobacco smoking	Decreased theophylline effect.

Some drugs are converted to toxic metabolites by drug metabolizing enzymes. Acetaminophen (paracetamol) is converted primarily to non-toxic metabolites, but small amount is converted to cytototoxic metabolite, N-acetyl benzoquinonimine. Enzyme inducers (such as alcohol) can increase the formation of the toxic metabolite and increase the risk of hepatotoxicity as well as damage to other organs (Snyder et al., 2012).

On the other hand, inhibition of metabolism can increase the effect/toxicity of the object drugs. Inhibitors of CYP3A4 enzymes increases the risk of toxicity from many drugs, including carbamazepine, cisapride, cyclosporine, ergot alkaloids, lovastatin, pimozide, protease inhibitors, rifabutin, simvastatin, tacrolimus, and vinca alkaloids.

Drugs that can inhibit non-microsomal enzymes are disulfiram, anticholinesterase agents, allopurinol, acetazolamide, MAOIs and metronidazole. Cimetidine (not ranitidine) reduces hepatic blood flow and thereby increases the bioavailability of propranolol. Propranolol also decreases both its own clearance and that of other drugs such as lignocaine. Other drugs that have the opposite effects increased blood flow through the liver so that the metabolism is increased (Brunton et al., 2017).

Table 4. Some examples of common drug interactions resulting from inhibition of hepatic microsomal enzymes

Drugs Affected	Enzyme Inhibitor	Effect of Interaction
Alcohol	Chlorpropamide, Metronidazole, Ketoconazole	Disulfiram like reaction due to rise in blood acetaldehyde
Oral anticoagulants	Metronidazole	Increased anticoagulant effect, bleeding tendency
Corticosteroids	Erythromycin	Increased corticosteroids effect, Toxicity possible
Phenytoin	Chloramphenicol, INH	Increased phenytoin level, Toxicity possible
Azathioprine	Allopurinol	Increased Azathioprine effect, increased toxicity

Excretion

The renal excretion of active drug can also be affected by the concurrent drug therapy. Certain drugs, weak acids or weak bases may be influenced by other drugs that affect urinary pH. This is due to changes in the ionization of the drug, thus altering the lipid solubility and the ability to be reabsorbed back from the renal tubule (Snyder et al., 2012).

Interference with reabsorption by the renal tubule can occur when there is alteration in the urinary pH. Alkalization of urine may increase the excretion of acidic drugs like salicylate in overdose and acidification may increase the excretion of basic drugs like amphetamine and quinine in acute overdose (Caterina et al., 2013).

Interference with active transport of organic acids across the renal tubular epithelium is seen with probenecid competing with penicillin. Interference with renal excretion of methotrexate by aspirin, zivovudine by probenecid and of digoxin by quinine, contributes to the potentially harmful interactions with these combinations.

Changes in kidney blood flow is partially controlled by the production of renal vasodilatory prostaglandins and when this synthesis is decreased by indomethacin, the renal excretion of lithium will be reduced and serum levels may rise as a result (Brunton et al., 2017; Snyder et al., 2012)

Pharmacodynamic Drug Interactions

With pharmacodynmics, there can be three types of interactions: additive, synergistic, and antagonistic. Additive or synergistic interaction occurs when two or more drugs with similar pharmacodynamic effects are given together. The additive or synergistic effects may result in excessive response and toxicity (Moses & McGuire, 2010; Brunton et al., 2017; Snyder et al., 2012).

Additive Interaction

Additive interaction means the effect of two chemicals is equal to sum of effect of two chemicals taken separately (usually due to two chemicals acting the same way. e.g., alcohol and depressants, tranquilizer, and painkillers).

Synergistic Interaction

Synergistic interaction means the effect of two chemicals is more than sum of separate effect at same doses (e.g., pesticide and fertilizers). Some examples are given in Tables 5 and 6.

Table 5. Common drugs causing synergistic effects due to interaction between the drugs

Drug 1 (Object)	Drug 2 (Precipitant)	Effects (Interaction)
CNS depressants	Drugs causing CNS depression	More CNS depression
Impramine	Phenelzine	Atropine-like poisoning
Mepyramine	Alcohol	More CNS depression causing accidents at work, machinery, road- traffic accidents
Anticholinergics	Antihistamine	Increased risk of anti-muscarinic side effects
Warfarin	Aspirin	Risk of bleeding
Aminoglycosides	Loop diuretics, Polymyxin	Nephrotoxicity, ototoxicity
Sulphonamides	Trimethoprim, Pyrimethamine	Sequential blockade
Methotrexate	Co-trimoxazole	Bone marrow megaloblastosis due to folic acid antagonist
Neuromuscular blockers	Drugs with neuromuscular blocking effect (aminoglycosides)	Increased neuromuscular blockade, delayed recovery, prolonged apnea
Potassium supplements, ACEI	Potassium sparing diuretics (Triamterine)	Marked hyperkalemia

Antagonistic Interaction

Antagonistic interaction occurs when drugs with opposing effects reduce the response to one or both drugs. Antagonistic interaction means effect of two chemicals is less than the sum of effect of two drugs taken independently (because the 2nd chemical increases excretion of 1st, or even directly blocks its toxic actions). Drugs that tend to increase blood pressure (such as nonsteroidal anti-inflammatory drugs) may inhibit the antihypertensive effect of drugs such as ACE inhibitors. Another example would be inhibition of response to benzodiazepines by concurrent use of theophylline (Snyder et al., 2012).

Not all drug interactions are bad. Some pharmacodynamics interactions occur directly on the receptor sites and provide beneficial effects. Some examples include naloxone for opiate (morphine) overdose, atropine for organophosphorous poisoning, isopreanline for beta-blocker overdose. Thus, antagonism forms the basis for antidotes of poisonings (Brunton et al., 2017; Snyder et al., 2012).

Table 6. Common drugs causing antagonistic effects due to interaction between the drugs

Drug 1 (Object)	Drug 2 (Precipitant)	Effects (Interactions)
Anticoagulants	Vitamin K	More CNS depression
Hypnotics	Caffeine	Decreased hypnosis
Oral Hypoglycemic Agents	Glucocorticocoids, Thiazides	Reduced hypoglycemic effects
Levodopa	Pyridoxine	Antagonize effect of Levadopa
Levodopa	Chlorpromazine	Each antagonize the effect of another (Anti-parkinsonism, anti- psychotic effect is reduced)
Antihypertensive agents	NSAIDs, Corticosteroids, Oral Contraceptives, Carbenoxolone	Decreased hypotensive effect due to salt and water retention
Thiazides, Furosemide	NSAIDs	Reduced diuretic effect due to salt and water retention
Sucralfate	Cimetidine, Sodium bicarbonate	Increased gastric pH prevents activation of sucralfate into gel

Some interactions can also occur outside the body, like mixing carbenicillin and gentamicin in a syringe can inactivate gentamicin.

DRUG-HERB INTERACTIONS

Herbal products are popularly used as complementary alternative medicines (CAM) worldwide for health promotion or treatment of various chronic diseases. Many patients take herbal products in combination with prescribed drugs without doctors' advice and most are unaware that combined ingestion of herbs with drugs may raise potential of herb drug interactions (Fasinu et al., 2012). Drug-herb interactions may be significantly under-reported and under-estimated and may probably be more frequent than drug–drug interactions because most patients (~70%) do not reveal their herbal use to their doctors (Thomson et al., 2012; Berman, 2001). Since herbal products are not scrutinized by the FDA as drugs, there is often a lack of comprehensive surveillance system for monitoring the adverse effects of herbs and drug. For most reported herb-drug interactions, due to paucity of literature and multiple ingredients involved, mechanisms involved in such interactions are often unknown. Since herbs can be seen as both a drug (Christensen et al., 2017). as well as food, altered drug absorption, metabolism, and clearance by active ingredients in combination may play a critical role in these interactions.

Many herbs can induce or inhibit liver and intestinal drug metabolizing enzymes (e.g., cytochrome P450s), leading to altered drug concentration and clearance. Reports of herbal products containing St John's Wort interacting with cyclosporine, amitriptyline, digoxin, indinavir, nevirapine, oral contraceptives, theophylline, simivastatin. Others include garlic supplements interacting with saquinavir; licorice increasing plasma concentration of prednisolone are some examples (Moses & McGuire, 2010).

Table 7. Some examples of common interactions occurring between herb and drugs

Herb	Common Usage	Drug(s)	Likely Interactions
St. John's Wort	Depression, mood stabilization	Cyclosporines, oral contraceptives, protease inhibitors	Can diminish effectiveness of cyclosporine. May compromise effectiveness of oral contra- ceptives, may lead to worsening symptoms for people with HIV taking protease inhibitors
Ginkgo	Memory improvement	Aspirin, anticoagulents	Can cause bleeding and hemorrhage
Kava	Anxiety	Alcohol, barbiturates, benzodiazepines	May enhance the effect and cause drowsiness or sedation
Ginseng	Athletic, improve sexual performance, boost immunity	Insulin, anticoagulants, antidepressants	May increase hypoglycemic effect of insulin. Can cause mania with antidepressants. Interfere with anticoagulants such as warfarin.

DRUG-FOOD INTERACTIONS

Food can influence bioavailability of drugs, which can be either acute (when a drug is taken with meal) or chronic (when the regularly consumed food items influence the drug absorption). Nature of interactions with food are complicated, varying with quantity (amount) and composition of the food (fatty meal); and the drug and its formulation (Brunton et al., 2017). Although the effect of food is not clinically important for many drugs, there are food-drug interactions which may have adverse consequences. Some drugs have strict guidelines about when to be taken in relation to meals. Generally, patients should be advised to take their medicines consistently at the same time with respect to meals. Understanding possible clinical implications of taking medicines with or without food is important for achieving quality use of medicines and health professionals must be able to advise patients about how medicines should be taken in relation to meals (Debnath et al., 2017). How food interact with drugs can be classified into 5 categories: causing reduced, delayed, increased, and accelerated absorption, changing drug bioavailability and those in which food has no effect.

- **Gastric Emptying:** Food delays gastric emptying and generally rate of absorption of drugs are slower. Extent of absorption is unchanged except with high fatty meals enhancing absorption through better dissolution of poorly soluble drugs (griseofulvin, halofantrine). Solutions and suspensions are less prone to interactions while enteric coated drugs are more susceptible. Drug chelation: drug interacting with food constituents such as tetracyclines and dietary calcium, penicillamine and heavy metal ions, iron formulations and tannic acid.
- **Changes in Drug Metabolizing Enzymes:** Food affecting hepatic or gut wall drug metabolizing enzymes (isoenzyme CYP3A4) seen with grapefruit and/or grapefruit juice, brassica vegetables (sprouts, cabbage, broccoli, cauliflower); aflatoxin B1 (lowering activity of UDP glucuronyl transferase/ glutathione S transferase); ethanol and paracetamol (enzyme induction).
- Changes in splanchnic blood flow and plasma protein binding as seen with beta-blockers (propranolol, metoprolol, labetalol) and hydralazine.

Thus, provision of timely and appropriate advice about the possible effects of meals on medicines should be practiced (Snyder et al., 2012).

DRUG-DISEASE INTERACTIONS

Many diseases have been known to alter the response of drugs and can again be classified as previously under pharmacokinetics and pharmacodynamics. Gastrointestinal diseases, like Crohn's pancreatic diseases (steatorrhea) can alter the gastric emptying time. Cardiac failure can lead to decreased absorption, altered volume of distribution, and decreased renal elimination. Renal diseases can decrease excretion and increased level of drugs in the blood as well as prolong the action of drugs. Liver diseases can decrease the inactivation or decrease activation of prodrugs, decrease the plasma protein for binding, decrease hepatic extraction (first pass effect and liver blood flow). Increased drug metabolism is seen in hyperthyroidism (Schmidt-Mende et al., 2019).

Although dramatic advances have been made in the study of drug interaction mechanisms over the past few decades, many of the interactions remain unsolved. The reason for unexplained interactions may be due to the fact that in some drug-drug interactions, more than one mechanism explained above may be occurring simultaneously (Brunton et al., 2017; Snyder et al., 2012).

SOLUTIONS AND RECOMMENDATIONS

Controlling Drug Interactions

Knowing how drug interactions occur, recognizing when it occurred and how to manage them is an important part of clinical practice of every practitioner, whether he may be allopathic or traditional. Patients taking several different medicines, seeing more than one physician, or having multiple health conditions should be made aware of drug interactions to avoid potential problems (Snyder et al., 2012). Nurses and pharmacists should ask the patient about all the over the counter (OTC) and prescription drugs, dietary supplements, vitamins, botanicals, minerals, and any herbals taken. Different OTC drugs may contain a combination with one or more of the same active ingredients. Attention should be paid to active ingredients in the products to avoid overdose. Drug interaction warnings are included in the actual product label and should be reviewed when using certain OTC drug products. Drug interactions are usually preventable and health professionals should evaluate the potential of their occurrence and initiate appropriate prevention or management strategies (Brunton et al., 2017).

The potential for clinically important drug interactions can often be predicted based on the drug properties, method of drug administration, and patient-specific parameters. Patients should be observed and monitored for adverse drug effects, particularly after a change in treatment; some interactions (e.g., effects that are influenced by enzyme induction) may take more than a week to appear. Consequently, adverse drug effects resulting from drug interactions can be prevented by making patient- and situation-specific assessments, avoiding concomitant administration by implementing alternative therapeutic strategies, or taking precautionary measures such as dosage adjustments and increased monitoring. Determining the most appropriate alternative medication requires careful consideration of patient-specific risks and benefits (Snyder et al., 2012).

Preventing Drug Interactions

Hearing patient's complaints can help alert the physician to identifying previously unreported reactions (Snyder et al., 2012). Famous interactions should be memorized and form the basis of a broader understanding of drug interactions in general by:

- Grouping medications (classification) allows one to extrapolate known data to a certain extent across drug groups.

- Asking patients to bring all drugs they have in a brown bag (Brown Bag Review) and checking for drugs that can interact adversely (MIMS Malaysia, identifying and preventing medication errors).
- Asking patients if they take alcohol, traditional medicine, or nutrient supplements (Vitamins, minerals, amino acids, and herbs or botanicals esp., St. John's Wort, vitamin E, ginseng and Ginko biloba) – check or advise not to take.
- Asking patients about drugs they are taking (especially the OTC medicines), what purpose, how they take, for how long, prescribed or self, or taking medications as directed.
- Providing information about all drugs they are taking, discarding the expired, not needed or not taking, making aware the most serious/frequent drug interactions that can occur with the medications that patient is taking.
- Asking the patient about the pharmacy the drugs were purchased (single pharmacy or multiple pharmacies).
- Asking patients to buy from single pharmacy, to ask pharmacist to keep list of medications bought regularly (up-to-date personal medication record), asking drug information for each purchase (how to take, food?) and to explain about any adverse effect to be expected. This prevents medication errors due to bad doctor handwriting, or similar drug names, changing brands, building good relationships with the pharmacist, provide better compliance. If the patient is hospitalized, always check the wrist band.
- Software checkers for drug interactions are widely available, and can be applied when using high alert drugs, drugs with narrow therapeutic index, or when new drugs are prescribed (http://reference.medscape.com/drug-interactionchecker).

CONCLUSION

Clinicians and nurses should know all their patients' current drugs, including drugs prescribed by other clinicians, as well as by Traditional Medicine Practitioners including all over-the-counter drugs, herbal products, and nutritional supplements and vice versa (Brunton et al., 2017). Asking patients relevant questions about diet and alcohol consumption is recommended. The fewest drugs in the lowest doses for the shortest possible time should be prescribed. The effects, desired and undesired, of all drugs taken should be determined because these effects usually include the spectrum of drug interactions. If possible, drugs with a wide safety margin should be used so that any unforeseen interactions do not cause toxicity. Thus, all health care professionals should minimize such risks by accurate management (dose adjustment, spacing of dosing times, and close monitoring of therapy) in drug combinations. If dosage adjustment is ineffective, the drug should be replaced by one that does not interact with other drugs being taken (Caterina et al., 2013).

REFERENCES

Berman, B.M. (2001). Complementary medicine and medical education. *BMJ, 322*(7279), 121–122.

Brunton, L., Knollmann, B., & Hilal-Dandan, R. (2017). *Goodman and Gilman's, The Pharmacological Basis of Therapeutics* (13th ed.). McGraw-Hill.

Caterina, P., Antonello, D. P., Chiara, G., Chiara, C., Giacomo, L., & Antonio, S. (2013). Pharmacokinetic drug-drug interaction and their implication in clinical management. *Journal of Research in Medical Sciences, 18*, 601–610. PMID:24516494

Catto, G., Cork, N., & Williams, G. (2014). Should medical students be taught alternative medicine? *British Medical Journal, 348*(g2417), 1–3. doi:10.1136/bmj.g2417 PMID:24682533

Christensen, C. M., Morris, R. S., Kapsandoy, S. C., Archer, M., Kuang, J., Shane-McWhorter, L., Bray, B. E., & Zeng-Treitler, Q. (2017). Patient needs and preferences for herb-drug-disease interaction alerts: a structured interview. *BMC Complementary and Alternative Medicine, 17*, 272. doi:1630-6 doi:10.1186/s12906-017-

Committee for Human Medicinal Products. (2012). *Guideline on the investigation of drug interactions.* European Medicines Agency, Science Medicines Health.

Debnath. S., Tejovathi. R., Babu. N. & Kumar. T. H. H (2017). An Overview on Food & Drug Interactions. *Pharma Times, 49*, 4.

Fasinu, P. S., Bouic, P. J., & Rosenkranz, B. (2012). An overview of the evidence and mechanisms of herb–drug interactions. *Front. Pharmacol, 3*(69).

Frenkel, M., Ben-Arye, E. & Hermoni, D. (2004). An approach to educating family practice residents and family physicians about complementary and alternative medicine Complement. *Ther. Med., 12*(2-3), 118-25.

Gabay, M., & Spencer, S. H. (2021). Chronic Conditions and Public Health. *PSAP, 3.* https://www.accp.com/docs/bookstore/psap/p2021b3_sample.pdf

Gray, A. C., Steel, A., & Adams, J. (2019). A critical integrative review of complementary medicine education research: Key issues and empirical gaps. *BMC Complementary and Alternative Medicine*, *19*(1), 73. doi:10.118612906-019-2466-z PMID:30894151

Kennedy, D. R. (2019). Redesigning a Pharmacology Course to Promote Active Learning. *American Journal of Pharmaceutical Education*, *83*(5), 6782. doi:10.5688/ajpe6782 PMID:31333258

Kumar-Pal, S. (2002). Complementary and alternative medicine: An overview. *Current Science*, *82*(5), 513–524.

Lecture Notes on Pharmacology. (2011). *Department of Medical Sciences, University of Pharmacy* (3rd ed.). Ministry of Health, Union of Myanmar.

Mann, D., Gaylord, S., & Norton, S. K. (2004). *Integrating Complementary & Alternative Therapies with Conventional Care. Program on Integrative Medicine.* University of North Carolina at Chapel Hill. http://pim.med.unc.edu

Moses, G. M., & McGuire, T. M. (2010). Drug interactions with complementary medicines. *Australian Prescriber*, *33*(6), 181. doi:10.18773/austprescr.2010.084

Page, C., Hoffman, B., Curtis, M., & Walker, M. (2006). *Integrated Pharmacology* (3rd ed.). Mosby Ltd.

Rao, A., Shakeel, M., Trinidade, A., Rao, G., Pearce, A., & Ah-See, K-M. (2012). The Importance of Complementary and Alternative Medicine Education in Medical School. *Journal of Evidence-Based Complementary & Alternative Medicine,* 1-7. doi doi:10.1177/2156587212451597

Schmidt-Mende, K., Andersen, M., Wettermark, B., & Hasselstrom, J. (2019) Drug–disease interactions in Swedish senior primary care patients were dominated by non-steroid anti-inflammatory drugs and hypertension – a population-based registry study. *Scandinavian Journal of Primary Health Care, 38*(3), 330-339. https://doi.dtorg/10.1080/02813432.2020.1794396

Smith, S., Newhouse, J. P., & Freeland, M. S. (2009). Income, insurance, and technology: Why does health spending outpace economic growth? *Health Affairs (Project Hope)*, *28*(5), 1276–1284. doi:10.1377/hlthaff.28.5.1276 PMID:19738242

Snyder, B. D., Polasek, T. M., & Doogue, M. P. (2012). Drug interactions: Principles and practice. *Australian Prescriber*, *35*(3), 85–88. [REMOVED HYPERLINK FIELD] doi:10.18773/austprescr.2012.037

Soliman. M. & Bilszta. J. L. (2021). Teaching complementary and alternative medicine in undergraduate medical education: a scoping review. *International Journal of Medical Education, 12,* 140-149. doi:10.5116/ijme.60e2.f3ed

Templeman, K., Robinson, A., & McKenna, L. (2015). Integrating complementary medicine literacy education into Australian medical curricula: Student-identified techniques and strategies for implementation. *Complementary Therapies in Clinical Practice, 21,* 238-246.

Thomson, P., Jones, J., Evans, J. M., Stephen, L., Leslie, S. L. (2012). Factors influencing the use of complementary and alternative medicine and whether patients inform their primary care physician. *Complementary Therapies in Medicine, 20*(1–2), 45-53. https://doi.org/10.1016/j.ctim.2011.10.001

Tiralongo, E., & Wallis, M. (2008). Integrating Complementary and Alternative Medicine Education into the Pharmacy Curriculum. *American Journal of Pharmaceutical Education, 72*(4), 74. doi:10.5688/aj720474 PMID:19002274

World Health Organization. (2019). *WHO global report on traditional and complementary medicine 2019.* World Health Organization. https://apps.who.int/iris/handle/10665/312342

Chapter 2
Food-Drug Interactions:
Types, Causal Mechanisms, Potential Consequences, and Preventive Strategies

Muhammad Adil
University of Veterinary and Animal Sciences Lahore, Jhang, Pakistan & Jhang Campus, Pakistan

Muhammad Asif
DHQ Teaching Hospital, Mardan, Pakistan

EXECUTIVE SUMMARY

Bioactive dietary ingredients can influence the pharmacokinetic and/or pharmacodynamic attributes of drugs that are orally administered either in conjunction with food or following a short interval. The pharmacokinetic form of food-drug interactions is reflected by changes in the rate/extent of drug absorption, distribution, metabolism, or excretion. Whereas, diet-induced pharmacodynamic modulation may arise in terms of additive, synergistic, or antagonistic effects. Most of the clinically important, food-drug interactions occur on account of altered drug bioavailability attributed to dietary constituents. Depending upon their occurrence and severity, food-drug interactions leading to enhanced plasma drug concentrations may have beneficial or harmful consequences. The outcomes of food-drug interactions may range from the loss of drug efficacy and subsequent treatment failure to serious adverse effects. Proper adherence to the drug-specific prescribing guidelines and patient compliance are requisite for minimizing the likelihood of potential food-drug interactions.

DOI: 10.4018/978-1-6684-7828-8.ch002

INTRODUCTION

Food-drug interactions can be defined as the biological, chemical or physiological interference between dietary substances and drugs (Genser, 2008; Santos & Boullata, 2005). A food-drug interaction may involve variation in the biodisposition or biological effects of drug(s) or concurrently used dietary substance(s). Similar to drugs, every food item does not essentially provoke the food-drug interactions. Despite the significance of food for the life and well-being of humans, the intake of certain food items along-with medication can cause potential food-drug interactions. In addition to the use of food items for the fulfillment of nutritional requirements, food-based supplements are also consumed for the therapy of various disease conditions. Particularly, the utilization of bioactive food products is usually emphasized for the prevention of ageing, obesity, malignancy, and cardiovascular disorders. Despite considered as non-toxic on account of being natural, the dietary substances and food supplements can be of serious concern in the context of potential food-drug interactions. Concurrently used dietary substances may alter the response of a patient to diagnostic and therapeutic modalities.

The increasing diversity of therapeutic agents and dietary substances is expected to further augment the chances of food-drug interactions. Certain indigenous dietary substances and food supplements are traditionally utilized by the patients without their extensive screening for potential interactive effects with therapeutic agents (Amadi & Mgbahurike, 2018). Therefore, the progressively growing consumption of vegetable supplements and natural foods has raised serious concerns regarding the food-drug interactions, primarily in patients who are subjected to chronic medication (Choi & Ko, 2017). Food-drug interactions constitute an important aspect of prescribing guidelines, usually overlooked by the physicians (Sørensen, 2002). In addition to dietary aspects, the use of food supplements should also be taken into consideration while prescribing drugs for the patients. The rising world-wide consumption of food supplements for therapeutic purpose necessitate their appropriate toxicological screening and regulation of manufacturing as well as sale. Although, the rising popularity of complementary and alternative medical practices among the physicians and patients, accompanied by increased funding opportunities have relatively accelerated the availability of scientific data about the safety and efficacy of dietary supplements and allied therapies, the scarcity of experimental data regarding most of the dietary supplements and complementary therapies impedes their safe consumption along with typical drugs. This chapter outlines the major clinically-significant food-drug interactions in terms of classification, mechanisms, consequences and preventive strategies.

CLASSIFICATION AND CAUSAL MECHANISMS OF FOOD-DRUG INTERACTIONS

Physico-chemical or biological interplay between a dietary ingredient and a drug is referred to as a food-drug interaction. Since the outcome of a food-drug interaction arises either in terms of pharmacokinetic or pharmacodynamic variations, thus similar to drug-drug interactions and drug-herb interactions, the food-drug interactions are also broadly classified into two major types of pharmacokinetic food-drug interactions and pharmacodynamic food-drug interactions. Certain food products can modulate the biological effects of drugs via interfering with their physico-chemical properties or mechanisms of action. Such type of interactions involving the alteration of mode of action or biological effect of drug(s), by the concurrently used food item(s) are known as pharmacodynamic food-drug interactions. For instance, the anticoagulant effect of warfarin is reversed by the concurrent use of vitamin K_1-containing green leafy vegetables. Likewise, potassium-containing fruits including banana and orange may potentiate the hyperkalemic effect of renin-angiotensin-aldosterone system blockers and consequently lead to myocardial arrhythmia and even cardiac arrest (Choi & Ko, 2017).

Interactions involving the modulation of absorption, distribution, metabolism, or excretion of drugs by concomitantly used food products are known as pharmacokinetic food-drug interactions. Besides the alteration of gastrointestinal $_{P}H$, gastric emptying, splanchnic blood flow, density of gut microflora and bile secretion are other possible mechanisms through which food items may affect the absorption of concurrently used drugs. Pharmacokinetic food-drug interactions can also result from the alteration of transporter proteins and metabolizing enzymes implicated in governing the disposition kinetics of drugs. The oral absorption and consequent anticonvulsant effect of phenytoin is reduced on account of its binding with diet-containing proteins (Lourenço, 2001). Similarly, reduced absorption and lack of antimicrobial effect also occur due to strong affinities of fluoroquinolones and tetracyclines for dietary magnesium and calcium, respectively (Polk, 1989). Conversely, fat-containing foods enhance the absorption of lipophilic antiviral protease inhibitors (Tiec et al., 2005).

More recently, the food-drug interactions have been categorized into four distinct types (Chan, 2013; Genser, 2008). Interactions occurring during the mixing or administration of nutrients and drugs prior to their introduction into the human body are referred to as type I food-drug interactions. For example, enteral nutrition can cause the adsorption of levothyroxine with the tubing, impaired dissolution and subsequent hypothyroidism. Type II food-drug interactions arise following the enteral or oral co-administration of nutrients and drugs with subsequent alteration in the functions of metabolizing enzymes, carrier proteins or complex formation. For instance, the intestinal CYP_3A_4 enzyme and solute carrier family 22A (SLC22A) transporter proteins are inhibited by grapefruit juice and valproic acid-containing berries, respectively. Whereas, complex formation (chelation) occurs following the co-consumption of ciprofloxacin and calcium-containing food items. The interaction between tyramine-containing fermented foods and mono amine oxidase (MAO) inhibitor antidepressant drugs presents an example of type III food-drug interactions, wherein the altered metabolism of catecholamines may lead to hypertensive crisis. Modulation of tissue-specific transporter proteins and entero-hepatic circulation trigger the type IV food-drug interactions.

Complex formation, partitioning and adsorption are most usual mechanisms through which dietary substances can influence the bioavailability and pharmacological effect of co-administered drugs. Nutrients can compete with drug molecules for the sake of carrier proteins and metabolizing enzymes located in the gastrointestinal tract. Accordingly, the plasma concentration and metabolic conversion of drugs can be significantly affected leading to either therapeutic failure or appearance of detrimental effects. The induction or inhibition of metabolizing enzymes by dietary ingredients may reduce or prolong the duration of action of substrate drugs. Majority of the reported food-drug interactions arise due to modulation of cytochrome (CYP) P450 enzyme system (Bazzie et al., 2006). CYP_3A_4 is considered as the principal drug metabolizing enzyme involved in most of the documented food-drug interactions (Fujita, 2004). In addition to the nature and bioactivity of dietary products, the likelihood of food-drug interactions also depend upon the physico-chemical profile of drug as well as the gastro-intestinal physiology of patient (Custodio et al., 2008).

Clinically Significant Major Food-Drug Interactions

Food-drug interactions attributed to grapefruit juice have been extensively reported in the literature. Grapefruit juice increases the bioavailability of nearly 40 different drugs due to its inhibitory effect on the intestinal CYP_3A_4 enzyme (Saito et al., 2005). Hepatic CYP_1A_2 and CYP_3A_4 are inhibited by apigenin, naringenin and flavonoids contained in grapefruit juice (Doostdar et al., 2000). Dermatologic toxicity occurred following the long-term simultaneous use of grapefruit juice and antineoplastic drug, docetaxel. However, two weeks after the discontinuation of grapefruit juice consumption by the patient, the plasma concentration of docetaxel returned to normal and resultant toxicity was subsided (Valenzuela et al., 2011). Likewise, marked QT prolongation resulting from the co-administration of grapefruit juice and amiodarone has been linked with the onset of ventricular arrhythmia (Agosti et al., 2012). Despite the inhibition of CYP_3A-mediated first-pass metabolism by the grapefruit juice, the half-life of affected drug still remained unaltered (Hanley et al., 2011). Moreover, the regular consumption of grapefruit juice had no appreciable impact on the half-life of intravenously administered midazolam (Kupferschmidt et al., 1995). Furanocoumarins have been identified as the bioactive components responsible for causing grapefruit juice-induced, food-drug interactions. Adverse drug reactions attributed to the interaction of grapefruit juice with several types of drugs including statins, antineoplastic drugs (such as vinblastine), antiarrhythmic drugs, beta-blockers, angiotensin II receptor antagonists and calcium channel blockers have been previously documented (Ofer et al., 2005; Owira & Ojewole, 2010). Owing to the likelihood of reported adverse drug events, patients receiving any of the afore-mentioned drugs are recommended to avoid the utilization of grapefruit juice. Conversely, enhanced plasma concentrations and therapeutic effects of lovastatin and simvastatin leading to relatively lower risk of ischemic heart disease have been associated with the use of grapefruit juice (Wang & Klass, 2016). Grape fruit juice inhibited the biotransformation of cilostazol and gave rise to purpura in an old patient (Kirby & Unadkat, 2007). Several studies have linked the grapefruit juice-mediated inhibition of CYP_3A_4 enzyme with significant food-drug interactions. Grapefruit juice affects the oral absorption of drugs that are substrates of CYP_3A_4, p-glycoprotein and organic anion transporter protein (De Castro et al., 2007; Li et al., 2007).

An *in vitro* study has demonstrated the inhibition of cytochrome P450 enzymes by the principal furanocoumarin component of grapefruit juice, known as bergamottin (He et al., 1998). Moreover, flavonoids such as naringenin and naringin are other important constituents of grapefruit juice responsible for potential food-drug interactions. Even just 250 ml equivalent to a single glass of grapefruit juice is sufficient for enhancing the bioavailability of concomitantly administered drugs (Dasgupta, 2008). In contrast to the initial dose of grapefruit juice, its subsequent regular consumption for next 14 days had no impact on the pharmacokinetics of felodipine (Lundahl et al., 1998). Whereas, clinically significant grapefruit juice-drug interactions became quite unlikely when an interval greater than 24 hours was followed (Lilja et al., 2000). Additionally, the pharmacokinetics of several drugs including carbamazepine, saquinavir, diazepam, cyclosporine, itraconazole and verapamil were significantly affected by the co-administration of grapefruit juice (Bistrup et al., 2001; Fuhr et al., 2002; Garg et al., 1998; Gubbins et al., 2004; Kupferschmidt et al., 1998; Özdemir et al., 1998). Nevertheless, the co-consumption of grapefruit juice had no considerable impact on the pharmacokinetics of phenytoin, digoxin and indinavir (Becquemont et al., 2001; Kumar et al., 1999; Penzak et al., 2002), whereas, it reduced the bioavailability of fexofenadine by inhibiting the intestinal organic anion transporter proteins (Dresser et al., 2005). Therefore, grapefruit juice-mediated food-drug interactions and resultant therapeutic outcomes require thorough elucidation by means of future research studies.

Pomelo juice that closely resembles the grapefruit juice, is also known for increasing the bioavailability of cyclosporine and tacrolimus (Egashira et al., 2003;

Grenier et al., 2006). Pomelo juice enhanced the bioavailability of cyclosporine through the inhibition of p-glycoprotein, CYP_3A_4 or both (Grenier et al., 2006). However, the bioavailability of cyclosporine remained unchanged following the co-administration of cranberry juice. Furanocoumarins have been identified as the major bioactive components of pomelo juice. The interaction of pomegranate juice with carbamazepine and those of cranberry juice with nifedipine and warfarin have been associated with the inhibition of CYP_3A enzyme (Hidaka et al., 2005; Suvarna et al., 2003; Uesawa & Mohri, 2006). Similar to grapefruit juice, seville orange juice also contains bergamottin and can increase the bioavailability of felodipine upon concurrent administration (Malhotra et al., 2001). Besides, the bioavailabilities of aluminium and parvastatin were increased when the drugs were taken in conjunction with orange juice (Fairweather-Tait et al., 1994; Koitabashi et al., 2006). Alternatively, orange juice reduced the bioavailability of certain drugs such as simvastatin, fexofenadine, celiprolol and clofazimine (Kamath et al., 2005; Koitabashi et al., 2006; Lilja et al., 2004; Nix et al., 2004). Reduced oral absorption of celiprolol has been attributed to the bioactive constituent of orange juice, called hesperidin (Uesawa & Mohri, 2008). Cranberry juice impairs the biotransformation of warfarin through the inhibition of CYP_2C_9 enzyme. Additionally, leafy green vegetables are known for reducing the hypoprothrombinemic effect of warfarin (Walker et al., 1996).

Despite the infrequent reports on CYP_3A inhibition caused by alcoholic beverages (such as wine and beer) and tea, its clinical significance has not been established so far (Huang et al., 2008). Cruciferous vegetables, charcoal-broiled foods and smoking have been linked with the induction of drug metabolizing enzymes (Dasgupta, 2008). Diet containing lower carbohydrates but higher proteins, enhanced the clearance of theophylline and propranolol in treated patients (Fagan et al., 1987). The co-consumption of MAO inhibitors with tyramine-rich fermented foods including cheese, salami, shrimp paste, yogurt, ripped bananas and red wine may lead to overproduction of catecholamines and subsequent hypertensive crisis (Brown et al., 1989; Volz & Gleiter, 1998). Cigarette smoking enhanced the plasma concentration of clozapine and resulted in seizures due to the inhibition of CYP1 A2 enzyme (Prior et al., 1999).

Calcium and casein, the integral components of milk may reduce the bioavailability of ciprofloxacin (Pápai et al., 2010). Owing to their high affinity for calcium contained in the milk and resultant formation of calcium orthophosphate chelates, the oral absorption of tetracyclines is significantly decreased (Gurley & Hagan, 2003). Similarly, cow milk contains the xanthine oxidase enzyme and may impair the oral absorption of cytotoxic drug, mercaptopurine (de Lemos et al., 2007). An *in vivo* study documented increased bioavailability of ibuprofen following the utilization of carbonated drink, Coca cola (Kondal & Garg, 2003). Whereas, co-

consumption of carbonated drinks is known for enhancing the oral absorption of antifungal drug, amphotericin B. Caffeine-containing beverages and foods such as tea, carbonated drinks, coffee, candies, and chocolates may potentiate the adverse effects of theophylline and methylxanthine derivatives.

Piperine, the principal ingredient of black pepper also enhances the bioavailability of many drugs including rifampicin, phenobarbitone, propranolol, theophylline, cefotaxime, amoxicillin, and phenytoin through the inhibition of CYP_3A_4 and p-glycoprotein (Bano et al., 1991; Bhardwaj et al., 2002; Hiwale et al., 2002; Mujumdar et al., 1990; Pattanaik et al., 2006; Zutshi et al., 1985). The interaction of apple with fexofenadine and that of tangerine with nifedipine have been documented in the literature (Bailey et al., 1991; Rodríguez-Fragoso & Reyes-Esparza, 2013). Furthermore, mango interacts with verapamil, diclofenac, and midazolam (Rodeiro et al., 2008). Vegetables such as spinach and tomatoes have also been associated with potential food-drug interactions (Platt et al., 2010; Wang & Leung, 2010). Watercress enhances the plasma level of muscle relaxant, chlorzoxazone via the inhibition of CYP_2E_1 enzyme (Telang et al., 2009). Moreover, cholinesterase inhibition caused by Solanceous vegetables including eggplant, potatoes and tomatoes may enhance the duration of action of general anesthetics (Krasowski et al., 1997).

CONSEQUENCES AND PREVENTION OF FOOD-DRUG INTERACTIONS

The susceptibility of an individual to food-drug interactions depends upon several other factors including the physiological status, comorbidities, polypharmacy, compliance, dietary habits, and hepato-renal as well as cardiovascular functions (Schmidt & Dalhoff, 2002). Besides, the predictability and intensity of several food-drug interactions significantly vary on account of the idiosyncratic characteristics of individual patients. Substantial variations exist in the nature, intensity, and clinical significance of food-drug interactions. Therapeutic failure resulting from the reduced bioavailability of drugs such as bisphosphonates, indinavir and tetracyclines represent the most serious type of food-drug interactions. However, certain pharmacokinetic food-drug interactions are not essentially translated into clinically detectable outcomes. Conversely, food-drug interactions considerably enhance the bioavailability and resultant pharmacological effects of saquinavir, griseofulvin and albendazole (Schmidt & Dalhoff, 2002). While, the increased bioavailability caused by food-drug interaction may potentiate the toxicity of drugs having a narrow margin of safety such as halofantrine, carbamazepine, tacrolimus, and hydralazine. Besides, some food-drug interactions may lead to beneficial effects. For instance, the adverse effects of non-steroidal anti-inflammatory drugs (NSAIDs) and erythromycin are minimized by the use of these drugs along with food (Schmidt & Dalhoff, 2002).

The rising quality standards of medical facilities require appropriate strategies for the identification and avoidance of food-drug interactions by the healthcare providers. Rational and evidence-based prescribing, patient compliance and proper record keeping may help to minimize the probability of food-drug interactions. In some cases, the drugs with proven widespread potential for interacting with food ingredients can be substituted by more safer alternatives. Additional prescribing guidelines are requisite for elderly patients, those suffering from chronic diseases and pregnant women, on account of their higher susceptibility to adverse food-drug interactions. Moreover, the latest digital-health approaches including artificial intelligence-based data mining techniques can be employed for predicting the potential food-drug interactions (Roy et al., 2022). The dietary intake of patients can be regulated by means of mobile health applications and wearable devices. Several user-friendly and reliable online databases such as Drug.com, Medscape and WebMD are available for checking the likely food-drug interactions by the patients themselves (Roy et al., 2022). Proper consultation is essential for enabling the patient to avoid the con-consumption of drugs and dietary substances suspected for potential interactive effects (Spanakis et al., 2022). The medication and dietary patterns of patients should be appropriately evaluated by the health professionals for precluding any possible food-drug interaction (Amadi & Mgbahurike, 2018). Integrated efforts involving the physicians, pharmacists, nursing staff and care takers can help to overcome the incidence of unfavorable food-drug interactions in hospitalized patients.

CONCLUSION AND FUTURE PERSPECTIVES

Food-drug interactions exhibit considerable importance, especially in the evolving framework of personalized medicine (Roy et al., 2022). Unlike drugs, the dietary supplements usually do not undergo efficacy and safety evaluation using a vigorous premarketing validation process (Gardiner et al., 2008). The highly diverse phytochemical constituents of most dietary products confound their appropriate screening and ultimate identification of individual substances responsible for causing the food-drug interactions. Commercially available dietary supplements may demonstrate substantial variations in terms of potency and safety. In contrast to extensive literature on drug-drug interactions, both experimental and clinical data pertaining to food-drug interactions is relatively rare due to huge diversity in the composition of human diet. The currently available information on food-drug interactions is primarily derived from case reports and animal-based experimental studies or extrapolated from the existing pharmacological data (Gardiner et al., 2008). Despite the availability of scientific evidence for some treatments, the efficacy and safety assessment of most complementary therapies still requires placebo-controlled, clinical investigations. Moreover, the conduction of randomized controlled clinical trials seems problematic in case of some alternative therapies (Kantor, 2009). Therefore, data regarding the potential interactions of dietary substances and drugs, particularly in cases of chronic diseases, remains inconclusive.

The merging field of nutrigenomics can be applied to explore the interface between dietary substances and genomic factors for explicating the cellular and molecular basis of food-drug interactions. The database called "nutrichem" provides valuable information regarding the chemical constituents of plant-based dietary substances. Personalized nutritional strategies can be designed using the pharmacomicrobiome framework to alleviate the incidence of food-drug interactions (Roy et al., 2022). Current advances in bioinformatics and precision medicine can be exploited for future research on food-drug interactions. In addition to the well-reported food-drug interactions, there are certain cases exhibiting relatively insufficient theoretical information and consequently need to be rigorously addressed by means of clinical studies (Spanakis et al., 2022). Besides, the critical assessment of food supplements by international and regional regulatory organizations may substantially contribute to standardization and quality enhancement of these products. Access to reliable information resources regarding the safety and efficacy of dietary substances can significantly minimize the likelihood of potential food-drug interactions.

REFERENCES

Agosti, S., Casalino, L., Bertero, G., Barsotti, A., Brunelli, C., & Morelloni, S. (2012). A dangerous fruit juice. *The American Journal of Emergency Medicine, 30*(1), 248.

Amadi, C. N., & Mgbahurike, A. A. (2018). Selected food/herb–drug interactions: Mechanisms and clinical relevance. *American Journal of Therapeutics, 25*(4), e423–e433. doi:10.1097/MJT.0000000000000705 PMID:29232282

Bailey, D., Spence, J., Munoz, C., & Arnold, J. (1991). Interaction of citrus juices with felodipine and nifedipine. *Lancet, 337*(8736), 268–269. doi:10.1016/0140-6736(91)90872-M PMID:1671113

Bano, G., Raina, R., Zutshi, U., Bedi, K., Johri, R., & Sharma, S. (1991). Effect of piperine on bioavailability and pharmacokinetics of propranolol and theophylline in healthy volunteers. *European Journal of Clinical Pharmacology, 41*(6), 615–617. doi:10.1007/BF00314996 PMID:1815977

Bazzie, K. L., Witmer, D. R., Pinto, B., Bush, C., Clark, J., & Deffenbaugh, J. Jr. (2006). National survey of dietary supplement policies in acute care facilities. *American Journal of Health-System Pharmacy*, *63*(1), 65–70. doi:10.2146/ajhp050106 PMID:16373467

Becquemont, L., Verstuyft, C., Kerb, R., Brinkmann, U., Lebot, M., Jaillon, P., & Funck-Brentano, C. (2001). Effect of grapefruit juice on digoxin pharmacokinetics in humans. *Clinical Pharmacology and Therapeutics*, *70*(4), 311–316. doi:10.1016/S0009-9236(01)13478-8 PMID:11673746

Bhardwaj, R. K., Glaeser, H., Becquemont, L., Klotz, U., Gupta, S. K., & Fromm, M. F. (2002). Piperine, a major constituent of black pepper, inhibits human P-glycoprotein and CYP3A4. *The Journal of Pharmacology and Experimental Therapeutics*, *302*(2), 645–650. doi:10.1124/jpet.102.034728 PMID:12130727

Bistrup, C., Nielsen, F. T., Jeppesen, U. E., & Dieperink, H. (2001). Effect of grapefruit juice on Sandimmun Neoral® absorption among stable renal allograft recipients. *Nephrology, Dialysis, Transplantation*, *16*(2), 373–377. doi:10.1093/ndt/16.2.373 PMID:11158415

Brown, C., Taniguchi, G., & Yip, K. (1989). The monoamine oxidase inhibitor—Tyramine interaction. *Journal of Clinical Pharmacology*, *29*(6), 529–532. doi:10.1002/j.1552-4604.1989.tb03376.x PMID:2666453

Chan, L. N. (2013). Drug-nutrient interactions. *Journal of Parenteral and Enteral Nutrition*, *37*(4), 450–459. doi:10.1177/0148607113488799 PMID:23674575

Choi, J. H., & Ko, C. M. (2017). Food and drug interactions. *Journal of Lifestyle Medicine*, *7*(1), 1–9. doi:10.15280/jlm.2017.7.1.1 PMID:28261555

Custodio, J. M., Wu, C.-Y., & Benet, L. Z. (2008). Predicting drug disposition, absorption/elimination/transporter interplay and the role of food on drug absorption. *Advanced Drug Delivery Reviews*, *60*(6), 717–733. doi:10.1016/j.addr.2007.08.043 PMID:18199522

Dasgupta, A. (2008). Drug–Herb and Drug–Food Interactions. Handbook of Drug Monitoring Methods, 235-261.

De Castro, W. V., Mertens-Talcott, S., Derendorf, H., & Butterweck, V. (2007). Grapefruit juice–drug interactions: Grapefruit juice and its components inhibit P-glycoprotein (ABCB1) mediated transport of talinolol in Caco-2 cells. *Journal of Pharmaceutical Sciences*, *96*(10), 2808–2817. doi:10.1002/jps.20975 PMID:17542018 de Lemos, M. L., Hamata, L., Jennings, S., & Leduc, T. (2007). Interaction between mercaptopurine and milk. *Journal of Oncology Pharmacy Practice*, *13*(4), 237–240. doi:10.1177/1078155207080802 PMID:18045784

Doostdar, H., Burke, M. D., & Mayer, R. T. (2000). Bioflavonoids: Selective substrates and inhibitors for cytochrome P450 CYP1A and CYP1B1. *Toxicology*, *1*(144), 31–38. doi:10.1016/S0300-483X(99)00215-2 PMID:10781868

Dresser, G. K., Kim, R. B., & Bailey, D. G. (2005). Effect of grapefruit juice volume on the reduction of fexofenadine bioavailability: Possible role of organic anion transporting polypeptides. *Clinical Pharmacology and Therapeutics*, *77*(3), 170–177. doi:10.1016/j.clpt.2004.10.005 PMID:15735611

Egashira, K., Fukuda, E., Onga, T., Yogi, Y., Matsuya, F., Koyabu, N., Ohtani, H., & Sawada, Y. (2003). Pomelo-induced increase in the blood level of tacrolimus in a renal transplant patient. *Transplantation*, *75*(7), 1057. doi:10.1097/01.TP.0000058545.35041.BE PMID:12698101

Fagan, T. C., Walle, T., Oexmann, M. J., Walle, U. K., Bai, S. A., & Gaffney, T. E. (1987). Increased clearance of propranolol and theophylline by high-protein compared with high-carbohydrate diet. *Clinical Pharmacology and Therapeutics*, *41*(4), 402–406. doi:10.1038/clpt.1987.48 PMID:3829577

Fairweather-Tait, S., Hickson, K., McGaw, B., & Reid, M. (1994). Orange juice enhances aluminium absorption from antacid preparation. *European Journal of Clinical Nutrition*, *48*(1), 71–73. PMID:8200332

Fuhr, U., Müller-Peltzer, H., Kern, R., Lopez-Rojas, P., Jünemann, M., Harder, S., & Staib, H. A. (2002). Effects of grapefruit juice and smoking on verapamil concentrations in steady state. *European Journal of Clinical Pharmacology*, *58*(1), 45–53. doi:10.100700228-002-0436-7 PMID:11956673

Fujita, K.-i. (2004). Food-drug interactions via human cytochrome P450 3A (CYP3A). *Drug Metabolism and Drug Interactions*, *20*(4), 195–218. doi:10.1515/DMDI.2004.20.4.195 PMID:15663291

Gardiner, P., Phillips, R. S., & Shaughnessy, A. F. (2008). Herbal and dietary supplement-drug interactions in patients with chronic illnesses. *American Family Physician*, *77*(1), 73–78. PMID:18236826

Garg, S. K., Kumar, N., Bhargava, V. K., & Prabhakar, S. K. (1998). Effect of grapefruit juice on carbamazepine bioavailability in patients with epilepsy. *Clinical Pharmacology and Therapeutics*, *64*(3), 286–288. doi:10.1016/S0009-9236(98)90177-1 PMID:9757152

Genser, D. (2008). Food and drug interaction: Consequences for the nutrition/health status. *Annals of Nutrition & Metabolism*, *52*(Suppl. 1), 29–32. doi:10.1159/000115345 PMID:18382075

Grenier, J., Fradette, C., Morelli, G., Merritt, G. J., Vranderick, M., & Ducharme, M. P. (2006). Pomelo juice, but not cranberry juice, affects the pharmacokinetics of cyclosporine in humans. *Clinical Pharmacology and Therapeutics*, *79*(3), 255–262. doi:10.1016/j.clpt.2005.11.010 PMID:16513449

Gubbins, P. O., McConnell, S. A., Gurley, B. J., Fincher, T. K., Franks, A. M., Williams, D. K., Penzak, S. R., & Saccente, M. (2004). Influence of grapefruit juice on the systemic availability of itraconazole oral solution in healthy adult volunteers. *Pharmacotherapy: The Journal of Human Pharmacology and Drug Therapy*, *24*(4), 460–467. doi:10.1592/phco.24.5.460.33350 PMID:15098799

Gurley, B. J., & Hagan, D. W. (2003). Herbal and dietary supplement interactions with drugs. In J. J. Wolfe (Ed.), *Hand book of food-drug Interactions* (pp. 259–293). CRC Press.

Hanley, M. J., Cancalon, P., Widmer, W. W., & Greenblatt, D. J. (2011). The effect of grapefruit juice on drug disposition. *Expert Opinion on Drug Metabolism & Toxicology*, *7*(3), 267–286. doi:10.1517/17425255.2011.553189 PMID:21254874

He, K., Iyer, K. R., Hayes, R. N., Sinz, M. W., Woolf, T. F., & Hollenberg, P. F. (1998). Inactivation of cytochrome P450 3A4 by bergamottin, a component of grapefruit juice. *Chemical Research in Toxicology*, *11*(4), 252–259. doi:10.1021/tx970192k PMID:9548795

Hidaka, M., Okumura, M., Fujita, K.-i., Ogikubo, T., Yamasaki, K., Iwakiri, T., Setoguchi, N., & Arimori, K. (2005). Effects of pomegranate juice on human cytochrome p450 3A (CYP3A) and carbamazepine pharmacokinetics in rats. *Drug Metabolism and Disposition: the Biological Fate of Chemicals*, *33*(5), 644–648. doi:10.1124/dmd.104.002824 PMID:15673597

Hiwale, A., Dhuley, J., & Naik, S. (2002). Effect of co-administration of piperine on pharmacokinetics of beta-lactam antibiotics in rats. *Indian Journal of Experimental Biology*, *40*(3), 277–281. PMID:12635696

Huang, S. M., Strong, J. M., Zhang, L., Reynolds, K. S., Nallani, S., Temple, R., & Burckart, G. J. (2008). New era in drug interaction evaluation: US Food and Drug Administration update on CYP enzymes, transporters, and the guidance process. *Journal of Clinical Pharmacology*, *48*(6), 662–670. doi:10.1177/0091270007312153 PMID:18378963

Kamath, A. V., Yao, M., Zhang, Y., & Chong, S. (2005). Effect of fruit juices on the oral bioavailability of fexofenadine in rats. *Journal of Pharmaceutical Sciences*, *94*(2), 233–239. doi:10.1002/jps.20231 PMID:15570603

Kantor, M. (2009). The role of rigorous scientific evaluation in the use and practice of complementary and alternative medicine. *Journal of the American College of Radiology*, *6*(4), 254–262. doi:10.1016/j.jacr.2008.09.012 PMID:19327658

Kirby, B., & Unadkat, J. (2007). Grapefruit juice, a glass full of drug interactions? *Clinical Pharmacology and Therapeutics*, *81*(5), 631–633. doi:10.1038j.clpt.6100185 PMID:17438537

Koitabashi, Y., Kumai, T., Matsumoto, N., Watanabe, M., Sekine, S., Yanagida, Y., & Kobayashi, S. (2006). Orange juice increased the bioavailability of pravastatin, 3-hydroxy-3-methylglutaryl CoA reductase inhibitor, in rats and healthy human subjects. *Life Sciences*, *78*(24), 2852–2859. doi:10.1016/j.lfs.2005.11.006 PMID:16412477

Kondal, A., & Garg, S. (2003). Influence of acidic beverage (Coca-Cola) on pharmacokinetics of ibuprofen in healthy rabbits. *Indian Journal of Experimental Biology*, *41*(11), 1322–1324. PMID:15332505

Krasowski, M. D., McGehee, D. S., & Moss, J. (1997). Natural inhibitors of cholinesterases: Implications for adverse drug reactions. *Canadian Journal of Anaesthesia*, *44*(5), 525–534. doi:10.1007/BF03011943 PMID:9161749

Kumar, N., Garg, S., & Prabhakar, S. (1999). Lack of pharmacokinetic interaction between grapefruit juice and phenytoin in healthy male volunteers and epileptic patients. *Methods and Findings in Experimental and Clinical Pharmacology*, *21*(9), 629–632. PMID:10669910

Kupferschmidt, H. H., Fattinger, K. E., Ha, H. R., Follath, F., & Krähenbühl, S. (1998). Grapefruit juice enhances the bioavailability of the HIV protease inhibitor saquinavir in man. *British Journal of Clinical Pharmacology*, *45*(4), 355–359. doi:10.1046/j.1365-2125.1998.t01-1-00687.x PMID:9578182

Kupferschmidt, H. H., Ha, H. R., Ziegler, W. H., Meier, P. J., & Krähenbühl, S. (1995). Interaction between grapefruit juice and midazolam in humans. *Clinical Pharmacology and Therapeutics*, *58*(1), 20–28. doi:10.1016/0009-9236(95)90068-3 PMID:7628179

Li, Y., Jiang, X., Lan, K., Zhang, R., Li, X., & Jiang, Q. (2007). Pharmacokinetic properties of rosuvastatin after single-dose, oral administration in Chinese volunteers: A randomized, open-label, three-way crossover study. *Clinical Therapeutics*, *29*(10), 2194–2203. doi:10.1016/j.clinthera.2007.10.005 PMID:18042475

Lilja, J. J., Juntti-Patinen, L., & Neuvonen, P. J. (2004). Orange juice substantially reduces the bioavailability of the β-adrenergic–blocking agent celiprolol. *Clinical Pharmacology and Therapeutics*, *75*(3), 184–190. doi:10.1016/j.clpt.2003.11.002 PMID:15001969

Lilja, J. J., Kivistö, K. T., & Neuvonen, P. J. (2000). Duration of effect of grapefruit juice on the pharmacokinetics of the CYP3A4 substrate simvastatin. *Clinical Pharmacology and Therapeutics*, *68*(4), 384–390. doi:10.1067/mcp.2000.110216 PMID:11061578

Lourenço, R. (2001). Enteral feeding: Drug/nutrient interaction. *Clinical Nutrition (Edinburgh, Lothian)*, *20*(2), 187–193. doi:10.1054/clnu.2000.0155 PMID:11327750

Lundahl, J., Regårdh, C., Edgar, B., & Johnsson, G. (1998). The interaction effect of grapefruit juice is maximal after the first glass. *European Journal of Clinical Pharmacology*, *54*(1), 75–81. doi:10.1007002280050424 PMID:9591935

Malhotra, S., Bailey, D. G., Paine, M. F., & Watkins, P. B. (2001). Seville orange juice-felodipine interaction: Comparison with dilute grapefruit juice and involvement of furocoumarins. *Clinical Pharmacology and Therapeutics*, *69*(1), 14–23. doi:10.1067/mcp.2001.113185 PMID:11180034

Mujumdar, A., Dhuley, J., Deshmukh, V., Raman, P., Thorat, S., & Naik, S. (1990). Effect of piperine on pentobarbitone induced hypnosis in rats. *Indian Journal of Experimental Biology*, *28*(5), 486–487. PMID:2401524

Nix, D. E., Adam, R. D., Auclair, B., Krueger, T. S., Godo, P. G., & Peloquin, C. A. (2004). Pharmacokinetics and relative bioavailability of clofazimine in relation to food, orange juice and antacid. *Tuberculosis (Edinburgh, Scotland)*, *84*(6), 365–373. doi:10.1016/j.tube.2004.04.001 PMID:15525560

Ofer, M., Wolffram, S., Koggel, A., Spahn-Langguth, H., & Langguth, P. (2005). Modulation of drug transport by selected flavonoids: Involvement of P-gp and OCT? *European Journal of Pharmaceutical Sciences*, *25*(2-3), 263–271. doi:10.1016/j.ejps.2005.03.001 PMID:15911222

Owira, P. M., & Ojewole, J. A. (2010). The grapefruit: An old wine in a new glass? Metabolic and cardiovascular perspectives. *Cardiovascular Journal of Africa*, *21*(5), 280–285. PMID:20972517

Özdemir, M., Aktan, Y., Boydağ, B., Cingi, M., & Musmul, A. (1998). Interaction between grapefruit juice and diazepam in humans. *European Journal of Drug Metabolism and Pharmacokinetics, 23*(1), 55–59. doi:10.1007/BF03189827 PMID:9625273

Pápai, K., Budai, M., Ludányi, K., Antal, I., & Klebovich, I. (2010). In vitro food–drug interaction study: Which milk component has a decreasing effect on the bioavailability of ciprofloxacin? *Journal of Pharmaceutical and Biomedical Analysis, 52*(1), 37–42. doi:10.1016/j.jpba.2009.12.003 PMID:20053516

Pattanaik, S., Hota, D., Prabhakar, S., Kharbanda, P., & Pandhi, P. (2006). Effect of piperine on the steady-state pharmacokinetics of phenytoin in patients with epilepsy. *Phytotherapy Research: An International Journal Devoted to Pharmacological and Toxicological Evaluation of Natural Product Derivatives, 20*(8), 683–686. doi:10.1002/ptr.1937 PMID:16767797

Penzak, S. R., Acosta, E. P., Turner, M., Edwards, D. J., Hon, Y. Y., Desai, H. D., & Jann, M. W. (2002). Effect of Seville orange juice and grapefruit juice on indinavir pharmacokinetics. *Journal of Clinical Pharmacology, 42*(10), 1165–1170. doi:10.1177/009127002237991 PMID:12362932

Platt, K., Edenharder, R., Aderhold, S., Muckel, E., & Glatt, H. (2010). Fruits and vegetables protect against the genotoxicity of heterocyclic aromatic amines activated by human xenobiotic-metabolizing enzymes expressed in immortal mammalian cells. *Mutation Research/Genetic Toxicology and Environmental Mutagenesis, 703*(2), 90–98. doi:10.1016/j.mrgentox.2010.08.007 PMID:20713174

Polk, R. E. (1989). Drug-drug interactions with ciprofloxacin and other fluoroquinolones. *The American Journal of Medicine, 87*(5), S76–S81. doi:10.1016/0002-9343(89)90028-4 PMID:2686430

Prior, T. I., Chue, P. S., Tibbo, P., & Baker, G. B. (1999). Drug metabolism and atypical antipsychotics. *European Neuropsychopharmacology, 9*(4), 301–309. doi:10.1016/S0924-977X(98)00040-6 PMID:10422890

Rodeiro, I., Donato, M., Lahoz, A., Garrido, G., Delgado, R., & Gómez-Lechón, M. (2008). Interactions of polyphenols with the P450 system: Possible implications on human therapeutics. *Mini-Reviews in Medicinal Chemistry, 8*(2), 97–106. doi:10.2174/138955708783498131 PMID:18289092

Rodríguez-Fragoso, L., & Reyes-Esparza, J. (2013). Fruit/vegetable-drug interactions: Effects on drug metabolizing enzymes and drug transporters. *Drug Discovery*, 1-33.

Roy, R., Marakkar, S., Vayalil, M. P., Shahanaz, A., Anil, A. P., Kunnathpeedikayil, S., ... Sathees, S. (2022). Drug-food Interactions in the Era of Molecular Big Data, Machine Intelligence, and Personalized Health. *Recent Advances in Food Nutrition & Agriculture, 13*(1), 27–50. doi:10.2174/2212798412666220620104809 PMID:36173075

Saito, M., Hirata-Koizumi, M., Matsumoto, M., Urano, T., & Hasegawa, R. (2005). Undesirable effects of citrus juice on the pharmacokinetics of drugs: Focus on recent studies. *Drug Safety, 28*(8), 677–694. doi:10.2165/00002018-200528080-00003 PMID:16048354

Santos, C. A., & Boullata, J. I. (2005). An approach to evaluating drug-nutrient interactions. *Pharmacotherapy: The Journal of Human Pharmacology and Drug Therapy, 25*(12), 1789–1800. doi:10.1592/phco.2005.25.12.1789 PMID:16305298

Schmidt, L. E., & Dalhoff, K. (2002). Food-drug interactions. *Drugs, 62*(10), 1481–1502. doi:10.2165/00003495-200262100-00005 PMID:12093316

Sørensen, J. M. (2002). Herb–drug, food–drug, nutrient–drug, and drug–drug interactions: Mechanisms involved and their medical implications. *Journal of Alternative and Complementary Medicine (New York, N.Y.), 8*(3), 293–308. doi:10.1089/10755530260127989 PMID:12165187

Spanakis, M., Patelarou, E., & Patelarou, A. (2022). Drug-Food Interactions with a Focus on Mediterranean Diet. *Applied Sciences (Basel, Switzerland), 12*(20), 10207. doi:10.3390/app122010207

Suvarna, R., Pirmohamed, M., & Henderson, L. (2003). Possible interaction between warfarin and cranberry juice. *British Medical Journal, 327*(7429), 1454. doi:10.1136/bmj.327.7429.1454 PMID:14684645

Telang, U., Ji, Y., & Morris, M. E. (2009). ABC transporters and isothiocyanates: Potential for pharmacokinetic diet–drug interactions. *Biopharmaceutics & Drug Disposition, 30*(7), 335–344. doi:10.1002/bdd.668 PMID:19623673

Tiec, C. L., Barrail, A., Goujard, C., & Taburet, A.-M. (2005). Clinical pharmacokinetics and summary of efficacy and tolerability of atazanavir. *Clinical Pharmacokinetics, 44*(10), 1035–1050. doi:10.2165/00003088-200544100-00003 PMID:16176117

Uesawa, Y., & Mohri, K. (2006). Effects of cranberry juice on nifedipine pharmacokinetics in rats. *The Journal of Pharmacy and Pharmacology, 58*(8), 1067–1072. doi:10.1211/jpp.58.8.0007 PMID:16872553

Uesawa, Y., & Mohri, K. (2008). Hesperidin in orange juice reduces the absorption of celiprolol in rats. *Biopharmaceutics & Drug Disposition*, *29*(3), 185–188. doi:10.1002/bdd.603 PMID:18344215

Valenzuela, B., Rebollo, J., Pérez, T., Brugarolas, A., & Pérez-Ruixo, J. J. (2011). Effect of grapefruit juice on the pharmacokinetics of docetaxel in cancer patients: A case report. *British Journal of Clinical Pharmacology*, *72*(6), 978–981. doi:10.1111/j.1365-2125.2011.04052.x PMID:21692829

Volz, H.-P., & Gleiter, C. H. (1998). Monoamine oxidase inhibitors: A perspective on their use in the elderly. *Drugs & Aging*, *13*(5), 341–355. doi:10.2165/00002512-199813050-00002 PMID:9829163

Walker, S. E., Shulman, K. I., Tailor, S. A., & Gardner, D. (1996). Tyramine content of previously restricted foods in monoamine oxidase inhibitor diets. *Journal of Clinical Psychopharmacology*, *16*(5), 383–388. doi:10.1097/00004714-199610000-00007 PMID:8889911

Wang, H., & Leung, L. K. (2010). The carotenoid lycopene differentially regulates phase I and II enzymes in dimethylbenz [a] anthracene-induced MCF-7 cells. *Nutrition (Burbank, Los Angeles County, Calif.)*, *26*(11-12), 1181–1187. doi:10.1016/j.nut.2009.11.013 PMID:20400267

Wang, Y., & Klass, E. (2016). Grapefruit with your statin? *The American Journal of Medicine*, *129*(8), e159. doi:10.1016/j.amjmed.2016.03.015 PMID:27453391

Zutshi, R., Singh, R., Zutshi, U., Johri, R., & Atal, C. (1985). Influence of piperine on rifampicin blood levels in patients of pulmonary tuberculosis. *The Journal of the Association of Physicians of India*, *33*(3), 223–224. PMID:4044481

Chapter 3
A Study of Third-Semester Traditional Chinese Medicine Science Students

Yinuo Wang
Xiamen University Malaysia, Malaysia

EXECUTIVE SUMMARY

Pharmacology is an important and compulsory subject for undergraduate traditional Chinese medicine (TCM) science students. However, at this stage, the third semester TCM science students still have some misunderstanding and neglects about pharmacology. The research method was conducted by interviewing four undergraduate TCM science students who had graduated and were planning to gain their next degree in different fields in terms of pharmacology studies methods, application of pharmacology knowledge, and perceptions of pharmacology. The study found third semester undergraduate TCM science students had difficulties in learning pharmacology. However, the use of mnemonics, scenario simulation, literature writing and reading, etc. helped to motivate students and assisted in memorizing relevant knowledge points. Third semester TCM science students should pay attention to the study of pharmacology and find appropriate method in the meantime. In addition, educators and educational institutions are recommended to adjust teaching strategies according to students' status.

DOI: 10.4018/978-1-6684-7828-8.ch003

INTRODUCTION

Pharmacology has a comprehensive and mature theoretical system for the interpretation of drug interactions in the body and is also crucial for the investigation of drug mechanisms of action. It not only broadens the students' knowledge of physiology and pathology, but also provides a crucial initiation for their future research work. The course in pharmacology as a foundation course in the undergraduate period can also help students to better participate in future research programs in clinical medicine, basic medicine, pharmacy, chemistry, biological sciences, etc. According to statistics in 2018, adverse drug reactions due to medication errors cause or contribute to up to 2420 deaths per year in the UK (Elliott, 2018), which means that poor and weak knowledge of pharmacology is an important factor in this tragedy. For students of Traditional Chinese medicine (TCM) department, pharmacology is the breakthrough of Chinese herbs being used in the pharmaceutical field, but also a powerful weapon to make TCM scientization. For instance, Tu Youyou, the winner of the 2015 Nobel Prize in Physiology or Medicine, graduated from the Department of Pharmacy of Peking University and won the prize for her invention of the new antimalarial drugs that named artemisinin and dihydroartemisinic, which reflects the great value of pharmacology in the application of TCM. Nevertheless, the truth is that the passion of nowadays students for learning pharmacology is unable to match the value created by pharmacology. A large number of students ashamed that their cognitive system of pharmacology and pharmacology-related knowledge is not mature enough and their grasp of key points is not firm sufficiently for practical application in clinical or scientific research. In addition, the abuse of Chinese medicine and other types of drugs is an important issue that endangers human health. As pharmacology is a difficult and demanding interdisciplinary course, it is not easy for third-semester undergraduates to learn in this major, so it is important to find appropriate learning strategies and methods.

This paper is based on the practical experience of graduated TCM science undergraduate in their third semester of pharmacology during undergraduate period to explain effective methods of learning pharmacology and its implications for the future. The objective is to make students aware of the importance of pharmacology in their future research activity and clinical work, to motivate those students to devoted themselves into studying pharmacology. In addition, the article also includes the study methods from TCM science graduates contribute to pharmacology courses, as well as the recommendation to write papers in the related field of pharmacology, as well as suggestions for the formulation of study plans.

METHODOLOGY

The study is conducted to explore the adoption and variety of methods for studying pharmacology knowledge by graduated TCM science student in their third semester of study during undergraduate period, as well as the application of pharmacology concepts by the students involved and the future direction of research they will pursue. Interviews and content integration will also be conducted in terms of students' master's and doctoral application's situations and the degree of participation in projects with a need for pharmacology.

The survey included four undergraduate TCM science students who had graduated and were planning to do their master's and doctoral studies in the fields of metabolic disease pharmaceutical, bioengineering, clinical Traditional Chinese medicine, and clinical Western medicine. The study does not involve the use of any sensitive personal data or research content. All respondents provided informed consent prior to participation in the interviews. No intention is given to compare the performance of students from different programs, but the dispersion of future destinations is intended to provide qualitative differences relevant to all.

According to their undergraduate pharmacology period, the four respondents were asked about:

Study Methods of Pharmacology Course

·The mastery of undergraduate pharmacology knowledge of the participants (mainly judged by undergraduate GPA in pharmacology course, mastery of master or doctor's project-related pharmacological knowledge, the feedback of examinations and interviews for master's and doctoral programs, whether they had the habit of reading pharmacology-related literature during their undergraduate period, and whether they had written and published pharmacology papers during their undergraduate period. Since the interviewees did not want to disclose information about their specific GPA, only a brief description is provided).

The direction and application of pharmacology knowledge in the master and doctor's research project.

The degree of difficulty in applying pharmacology knowledge at the beginning of their future projects (including the difficulty in understanding the special pharmacology literature and the difficulty in understanding and writing the pharmacology mechanism in the related research projects)

Personal insights into undergraduate courses in pharmacology (mainly including the necessity of conducting relevant experiments in undergraduate course, importance of reading relevant literature in undergraduate course, importance of writing relevant pharmacology articles in undergraduate course)

Based on the above answers of questions to analyze the importance and necessity of pharmacology for undergraduates of Traditional Chinese medicine.

RESULTS

The Mastery of Undergraduate Pharmacology Knowledge of the Participants

GPA is the vital and intuitive reflection of relevant course knowledge assessment in undergraduate period.

The mastery of master or doctor's project-related pharmacological knowledge mainly shows students' understanding of the microscopic level theoretical knowledge of pharmacology in participating projects.

The feedback of participants in examinations and interviews for master's and doctoral programs mainly shows students' application and reserve of undergraduate pharmacology knowledge and the self-study ability in pharmacology area before entering their programs.

Whether the participants had the habit of reading pharmacology-related literature during their undergraduate period can be used as a reflection of participants' degree of emphasis on pharmacology and the learning enthusiasm during undergraduate study.

Whether participants had written and published pharmacology papers during their undergraduate period can reflect the practical application ability of participants' pharmacological knowledge to a certain extent.

Based on Table 1, Participant 3 had the best overall scores, and Participant 1 had a more evenly distributed score. Besides, the Participant 4 had a strong self-learning ability of pharmacological knowledge, and Participant 2 had a comprehensive grasp of project-related knowledge. It is means that each participant had different mastery of pharmacology knowledge and expertise in this area. In addition, every participant shows different degree of interests in pharmacology, and they had different bases of pharmacological knowledge.

The Direction and Application of Pharmacology Knowledge in the Master's and Doctoral Research Project

The application of pharmacology is extremely wide, and research often contains many pharmacological directions. The variety of application directions of pharmacology proves the importance of pharmacology in scientific research and clinical work. Its application is the embodiment of pharmacological work.

According to Table 2, although all participants are researchers in different projects, their projects contain a large amount of pharmacology knowledge, and pharmacology plays a crucial role for students in different fields.

The Degree of Difficulty in Applying Pharmacology Knowledge at the Beginning of Their Future Projects

Combined with the basic information of the four participants and the degree of difficulty in applying pharmacology knowledge at the beginning of their future project, it can be concluded that the mastery of basic knowledge of pharmacology and the reading and writing of pharmacological literature during undergraduate period are important for students' future development.

Personal Insights Into Undergraduate Courses in Pharmacology

The participants' own experiences are used to analyze the importance of the pharmacology curriculum and literature, and the direction of teaching.

According to the Table 4, it can be seen that all participants believe that pharmacology is essential to the future development of undergraduates in the department of TCM science, and that reading and writing pharmacological literature are extremely helpful. At the same time, pharmacological experiments are also advocated.

Study Methods of Pharmacology Course

Understand the Mechanism of Drugs by Watching Related-Pictures and Videos

A drug may act at the molecular level by altering the chemical structure of certain substances, through affecting upstream or downstream signaling pathways, or by combining its effects through multiple signaling or chemical pathways. For example, berberine which is a kind of Chinese herb extracts can target TAU proteins in Alzheimer's disease to exert its potential therapeutic effects on this kind of degenerative neural diseases, or it also has the ability to regulate ferroptosis via nrf2/GPX4. These pathways may seem tedious, but they are actually relevant to what TCM sciences students have learned in their undergraduate courses. The pictures and videos are more visual and easier for students to accept than the purely textual explanation of the mechanism. According to the feedback of participants, they indicated that in the process of learning pharmacology, they would tend to give up halfway through reading PPT and textbooks, and even it was difficult to focus on half an hour of recitation and reading pharmacological knowledge. Therefore, visualization of drug pathways is a recommended way to understand the knowledge points. For example, one of the participants liked drawing picture so the participant would retrieve a picture-based explanation of the signaling pathway through Google, and then draw the pathway simply by his own understanding. In this way, the upstream and downstream of the signaling pathway can be clearly distinguished, which part of a substance is involved in signaling, and the overall mechanism of action of the drug can be understood at a glance, and the pictures are more clearly imprinted on the students' brains than the dull words, which benefit student's response and memory for those pharmacological knowledge.

Aysha Rooha et al. published a cross-sectional study of children's short-term memory abilities in 2021 and concluded that pictures were more useful for children's short-term memory than words (Aysha Rooha, 2021). It is not a tedious mode of memorization, but rather it mobilizes the analytical ability of the self to deepen the memory of themselves through extensive reading and study of the pictures. In addition to picture-helped memorization, watching video lectures of relevant chapters is also an effective way to solve the problem. In pharmacology classes, our professor Dr. Aslam, often shares videos with us, which not only relieve the pressure of studying, but also explain more clearly the connection between drugs and human organs, even at the molecular level, such as the relationship between cells and receptors. This also provides a way for TCM science students to understand the pharmacokinetics of drugs.

Deepen the Understanding of Pharmacological Mechanisms by Reading the Relevant Literature

There are various types of literature, such as RCTs, clinical trials, and reviews. The students are recommended to choose a particular drug or therapeutic direction's Reviews to read in order to get a general idea of the progress of the entire drug or therapeutic area. These reviews often include descriptions of specific conditions, current mechanisms of the related drug, and so on. This is what the students need to memorize at the undergraduate period. In participants undergraduate years, their pharmacology professor once assigned an assignment to write a scoping review on diabetic foot and Traditional Chinese medicine, in which students not only mastered how to write a scoping review, but more importantly, their knowledge on the use of drugs for diabetic foot was expanded. Drug research in metabolic endocrine disorders is an important part of the medical field today, so it is beneficial for undergraduates to write a scoping review on this topic. In one of the participants cases, she has read at least 183 papers just in the process of writing this scoping review, in which the knowledge of both Chinese and Western medicines has been covered, and this is more conducive to understanding the content of the pharmacological course itself. The content of the related literature often includes experimental design, basic information of the experiment, drug usage, experimental results and so on. This type of comparison not only expands the students' knowledge of basic clinical or RCT experiments, but also grasps the contemporary understanding of the content consolidation and novel thinking about the drugs used to treat diabetic foot.

The pharmacological knowledge in the literature is more profound and relevant compared to textbooks. By writing and publishing a thesis, one can improve the competitiveness of future graduate applications, and the other can grasp the current research hot spots and collect information on some pharmacological studies. Third, it helps for the memory of drug-related pharmacokinetics and clinical applications. Fourth, it improves students' research interest in the direction of pharmacology and lays down future research directions. Fifth, to reduce the risk and harm caused by clinical errors in drug use. For example, both herbal and western drugs need to be dosed, and overdose has the danger to cause damage or even irreversible burden to organs inside human body. Therefore, in the course of pharmacology, the dosage of drugs is often discussed, and the memory of the dosage is often complicated and miscellaneous, which requires students to adopt a more flexible way of memory. In the process of exploring related literature, the concept of dosage is deepened, for example, the effect of ROS excess and deficiency on insulin resistance (Yadollah, 2014), one is oxidative stress and the other is the mechanism of reductive stress. In this case, the role of some herbs or herbal extracts is involved. For example, berberine, extracted from Huang Lian, may affect the phosphorylation of AMPK in the AdipoR-AMPK pathway by AdipoRon, as it may interfere with the application of ROS, which can be a positive and mitigating effect (Wei Li, 2020). In addition to describing the role of dosage, there are other embodiments of knowledge points emphasized in pharmacology textbooks in similar literature. For example, the role of receptors and molecular signaling pathways, oxidation and reduction reactions, and RAS are all emphasized in the literature. The memory of the different types of molecular pathways will be strengthened during repeated viewing of the relevant papers. Reading the literature may be boring at first, but once you find yourself less hindered by reading the literature, it means that you have a deeper understanding of how drugs work on the human body. According to participants personal observation, the quality of the thesis work is directly proportional to the degree of students' mastery of pharmacology knowledge. As a result, the writing and reading of literature is not only a publication task, but also a broadening of knowledge and an improvement of pharmacology-related cognition. At a superficial level, it can deepen students' memory of pharmacology knowledge, and at a deeper level, it is a crucial base for their future research direction in pharmacology.

The Use of Mnemonics

There are various mnemonic methods, such as Ebbinghaus forgetting curve, music mnemonic, smell mnemonic, emotional mnemonic, visual mnemonic, etc. The content of pharmacology is indeed a bit complicated for TCM science undergraduates. Therefore, students can use partial mnemonics to learn and remember the content. For example, the chapter on antibiotics was the hardest for TCM science undergraduates to remember. The contents of this chapter are huge and indispensable. For cephalosporins aspect alone, there are many kinds of drugs, most of which have similar spelling and have different preferences in function. It is necessary to categorize the antiseptic and antiviral as well as the antiparasitic, and to distinguish the different treatment routes before and after the infection. It is means that, for this kind of huge memory system, it is necessary to use mnemonics to assist. As an example, the Ebbinghaus forgetting curve (Murre, 2015) uses the pattern of human forgetting to efficiently remember complicated and miscellaneous contents.

Dialogue and Ask Each Other Related Questions

In the process of dialogue, people's thinking and reaction ability, visual and auditory ability are activated, which is helpful for students to use knowledge more flexibly, and in the setting of the situational dialogue, the students have to memorize the relevant lines, which are the tools for linking with the relevant pharmacological knowledge points. In the meantime, emotions are stimulated in situational dialogues, and it can enhance the subjective feeling of recall (independent from the correctness of memory), which can increase human confidence in memory. Vividness of memory for emotionally relevant events is often considered a marker of memory accuracy (Brosch, 2013). Enhancing the depth of students' memories of events through various dimensions would be more flexible and interesting than mere memorization. In the course of undergraduate pharmacology, the participants were once assigned a presentation that was for each of our groups to present the drug's introduction, and one of the groups spoke about the topic in a situational dialogue, which became a carrier conducive to mass recall both for themselves and their audience. For my students' private study, they are recommended to find a study partner in the process of studying pharmacology to optimize their memory by asking each other questions after the initial recitation of the PPT. Although this approach may take longer than direct memorization, it allows students to have a stronger grasp of knowledge. This also provides new ideas for the development of pharmacology teaching models, such as having students prepare a scenario that not only includes relevant pharmacology topics, but also allows both the listener and the speaker to gain a degree of emotional integration of the knowledge.

Actively Participate in Clinical Internship and Visit the Institute of Pharmacy

The clinical internship allows students to observe more clinical drug use and to gain a better understanding of pharmacodynamics as well as the commercial products of the corresponding drugs. In addition, the laboratory experience makes students to learn basic laboratory skills early, which is valuable for their future work as researchers. The study of pharmacology can be a useful tool to learn more about pharmacodynamic or pharmacokinetic theories of molecular pathways or receptor activation. In order to understand relevant pharmacological studies, students are often required to explore the pharmacology of specific drugs or diseases. For example, in Parkinson's and Alzheimer's neurological diseases, the pharmacology of the role of Lewy bodies, tau proteins, etc. needs to be explored. Even the latest research direction imparted by some institutes is to take the same prodrome of Parkinson's and COVID-19, which is heterosmia, and the same prodrome is used to analyze the neurological sequelae of COVID-19. This seems to be the domain of knowledge in physiology and pathology, but it is also the basis for pharmacological analysis of the mechanism of action of drugs in the human body. It is also one of the more breakthrough pharmacological learning methods to analyze possible drug treatment schemes by finding the same mechanism between different diseases.

CONCLUSION

In this paper, we integrate and discuss the methodology of pharmacology study for undergraduate Traditional Chinese medicine students. An interview study was conducted to analyze the knowledge and understanding of four TCM graduates with different program's directions in master or doctor's projects, to emphasize the importance and necessity of pharmacology study, and to explore the learning strategies and methods to provide appropriate teaching guidance and direction for educators and educational institutions. From this interview, it can be conclude that:

Among these four research directions, pharmacology plays an important role and cannot be ignored.

Traditional Chinese medicine undergraduates are generally not good at memorizing and mastering pharmacology courses, which is related to the different theoretical systems of Chinese and western medicine, but it is not insoluble.

The reading and writing of pharmacology related literature by TCM science undergraduates during their undergraduate period can help them formulate and develop their potential future research.

Pharmacological experiments and reading and writing of pharmacological literature are important for TCM science undergraduates to learn pharmacology and will be beneficial for the future.

Educators and educational institutions can promote pharmacological literature and experiments to assist students in learning pharmacology.

Students who have the habit of reading and writing pharmacological literature during their undergraduate period will adapt into their master's and doctoral projects better and faster, and will help them gain recognition from assessments.

People's inertia and avoidance can cause them to give up the pursuit of a slightly difficult but important thing. The difficulty of pharmacology course does exist for third semester TCM science undergraduates, which requires a good grasp of the basic theory of western medicine. However, it is naive to avoid pharmacology as a course that is important for both clinical and scientific research. On the contrary, students should try their best to master and understand the knowledge of this course, so as to better apply it in practice and lay the foundation for future research and knowledge system.

REFERENCES

Brosch, T., Scherer, K. R., Grandjean, D., & Sander, D. (2013). The impact of emotion on perception, attention, memory, and decision-making. *Swiss Medical Weekly, 143*, w13786. doi:10.4414mw.2013.13786 PMID:23740562

Elliott, R. Camacho, E. Campbell, F. Jankovic, D. Martyn St. James, M. Kaltenthaler, E. Wong, R. Sculpher, M. J., & Faria, R. (2018). Prevalence and Economic Burden of Medication Errors in the NHS in England. In *Rapid Evidence Synthesis and Economic Analysis of the Prevalence and Burden of Medication Error in the UK.* Policy Research Unit in Economic Evaluation of Health and Care Interventions Universities of Sheffield and York, Manchester, UK.

Li, W., Li, D., Kuang, H., Feng, X., Ai, W., Wang, Y., Shi, S., Chen, J., & Fan, R. (2020). Berberine increases glucose uptake and intracellular ROS levels by promoting Sirtuin 3 ubiquitination. *Biomedicine & Pharmacotherapy, 121*, 109563. doi:10.1016/j.biopha.2019.109563

Murre, J. M., & Dros, J. (2015). Replication and Analysis of Ebbinghaus' Forgetting Curve. *PLoS One, 10*(7), e0120644. doi:10.1371/journal.pone.0120644 PMID:26148023

Rooha, A., Anil, M. A., & Bhat, J. S. (2020). Pictures over words: A cross-sectional study reporting short term memory abilities in children. *F1000 Research*, *9*, 380. doi:10.12688/f1000research.23378.2 PMID:33520190

Yadollah, S., Kazemipour, N., Bakhtiyari, S., & Nazifi, S. (2017). Palmitate-induced insulin resistance is attenuated by Pioglitazone and EGCG through reducing the gluconeogenic key enzymes expression in HepG2 cells. *Journal of Medicine and Life*, *10*(4), 244–249. PMID:29362600

APPENDIX

Table 1. The Mastery of undergraduate pharmacology knowledge of the participants

Assessment Items Project of Participants	Metabolic Disease Pharmaceutical (Participant 1)	Bioengineering (Participant 2)	Clinical Traditional Chinese Medicine (Participant 3)	Clinical Western Medicine (Participant 4)
GPA of pharmacology course	Average	A little worse	Distinction	A little worse
The mastery of master or doctor's project-related pharmacological knowledge	·Mainly at the level of molecular pharmacology ·Project-related pharmacology knowledge was commanded meticulously and variously	Macro-pharmacology and molecular pharmacology are involved in a comprehensive grasp	It is mainly the clinical application of pharmacology. The theoretical knowledge reserve is extremely proficient, but the clinical application is slightly lacking	Mainly in the level of molecular pharmacology, for the direction of relevant pharmacology to master detailed and comprehensive
The feedback of participants in examinations and interviews for master's and doctoral programs	·Smooth ·Got the professor's recognition of knowledge reserve.	·Smooth ·No interviews	·Smooth ·Interview results are excellent	·Smooth ·The experimental design for the molecular diameter and cell injection of the traditional Chinese medicine extract is extremely careful, which is greatly praised by the professor
Whether the participants had the habit of reading pharmacology-related literature during their undergraduate period	Yes	Yes	No	No
Whether participants had written and published pharmacology papers during their undergraduate period	Yes	Yes	Yes	No

Table 2. The Direction and application of pharmacology knowledge in the master and doctor's research project

Assessment Items Project of Participants	Metabolic Disease Pharmaceutical (Participant 1)	Bioengineering (Participant 2)	Clinical Traditional Chinese Medicine (Participant 3)	Clinical Western Medicine (Participant 4)
Directions of application of pharmacology	·Molecular Pharmacology ·Anti-inflammatory and immunological pharmacology ·Clinical Pharmacology ·Quantitative pharmacology ·Metabolic disease pharmacology ·Pharmacokinetics ·Pharmacodynamics	·Molecular Pharmacology ·Quantitative pharmacology ·Pharmacokinetics ·Pharmacodynamics	·Renal pharmacology ·Clinical pharmacology ·Pharmacodynamics ·Pharmacology of Chinese materia medica	·Pharmacology of Chinese materia medica ·Clinical pharmacology ·Pharmacodynamics·Pharmacology of reproductive system diseases
Situation of application	Since this participant is a graduate student in pharmacy, the knowledge of pharmacology involved is extensive. That is to say, pharmacology plays an important role in this student's study project.	The experiments, research reports and papers involving drugs to reflect the relevant body reactions of mice in bioengineering need the support of pharmacological knowledge.	The application of herbs in the clinical diagnosis of traditional Chinese medicine needs to explore the influence of related Traditional Chinese medicine on the therapeutic effect of diseases through pharmacology.	Herb extracts are used in western medicine to target the treatment of related diseases. The molecular diameter of such extracts is closely related to the medicinal effect, and the mechanism of drug action is very important for research doctors.

Table 3. The degree of difficult in applying pharmacology knowledge at the beginning of their future projects

Assessment Items Project of Participants	Metabolic Disease Pharmaceutical (Participant 1)	Bioengineering (Participant 2)	Clinical Traditional Chinese Medicine (Participant 3)	Clinical Western Medicine (Participant 4)
Degree of difficulty in understanding specialized pharmacological literature	Due to the high requirement of pharmacological knowledge in the field of pharmacy, the participant found it very difficult to understand the relevant theories when he read the relevant literature at the beginning, but he could solve the problem and remember it through repeated retrieval and thinking.	Slightly difficult, can understand the general content, but the details need to be repeatedly searched. The mechanism of drug action is more difficult to understand.	Generally, can master specific content.	It's a little difficult. Detail points need to be retrieved repeatedly. Molecular pharmacology is more difficult to understand.
Difficulty in writing pharmacological mechanisms in relevant research plans	Skilled	Skilled	Not skilled	Not skilled

Table 4. Personal insights into undergraduate courses in pharmacology

Assessment Items Project of Participants	Metabolic Disease Pharmaceutical (Participant 1)	Bioengineering (Participant 2)	Clinical Traditional Chinese Medicine (Participant 3)	Clinical Western Medicine (Participant 4)
Whether pharmacology is considered important for students' future development	Yes	Yes	Yes	Yes
The importance of conducting relevant experiments in undergraduate course	Important	Important	Important	Important
Necessity of writing and reading relevant pharmacology articles in undergraduate course	Indispensable	Indispensable	Indispensable	Indispensable

Chapter 4
A Bio-Therapeutically Squalene:
Case Review for T&CM Students as a Wound-Healing Compound

Muhammad Shahzad Aslam
https://orcid.org/0000-0003-2728-6726
School of Traditional Chinese Medicine, Xiamen University Malaysia, Malaysia

Yun Jin Kim
https://orcid.org/0000-0001-8853-6587
School of Traditional Chinese Medicine, Xiamen University Malaysia, Malaysia

Qian Linchao
School of Traditional Chinese Medicine, Xiamen University Malaysia, Malaysia

EXECUTIVE SUMMARY

Although the skin tissue on our bodies is a well-organized structure with high biomechanical properties like tensile strength and friction, we have all experienced various types of wounds throughout our lives owing to numerous etiological factors. In the general population, it is a substantial source of morbidity. For instance, in the case of burnt skin tissue, self-healing is in fact a large and challenging barrier to tissue regeneration. Squalene is a bioactive triterpene that occurs naturally and plays a key role in the process of making sterols. The most well-known source of squalene is shark liver oil. Vegetable oils may contain squalene in a range of concentrations. They have been extracted using a variety of techniques, including supercritical carbon dioxide, microwave, ultrasonic, cold press, and traditional Soxhlet extractions. In vitro and in animal models, these substances have been demonstrated to have anticancer, antioxidant, drug carrier, detoxifier, skin moisturising, and emollient effects.

DOI: 10.4018/978-1-6684-7828-8.ch004

INTRODUCTION

Our body's skin tissue is a well-organized structure with good biomechanical qualities including tensile strength and friction but due to various etiological reason we all suffered from different kinds of wound in our life. It represents a significant cause of morbidity in the general population (Srinivasaiah et al., 2007). For-example, self-healing is indeed a significant and difficult barrier to tissue regeneration in the case of burnt skin tissue.

Squalene is a naturally occurring bioactive triterpene that serves as a crucial step in the production of sterols (Abuobeid et al., 2022). Shark liver oil is the best-known source of squalene (Rosales-Garcia et al., 2017). Squalene can be present in a variety of amounts in vegetable oils (Rotondo et al., 2017). They have been extracted in various methods such as supercritical carbon dioxide (He et al., 2003), microwave-assisted extraction (Lozano-Grande et al., 2019), ultrasonic-assisted extraction (Xiao et al., 2018), cold press technology (Akin et al., 2018) and conventional Soxhlet extractions (Ortega et al., 2012). These compounds have been shown to have anticancer (Owen et al., 2004), antioxidant (Sabeenafarvin et al., 2004), drug carrier (Couvreur & Vauthier, 2006), detoxifier, skin moisturising, and emollient properties both in animal models and in vitro settings (Kim & Karadeniz, 2012).

There are dozens of studies that indicate squalene as wound healing therapeutic agent in in-vitro cell line models and animals' model. Modern scaffolds play a significant role in tissue regenerative concepts in healing the burn skin. Squalene-loaded emulgel scaffold could be an effective formulation used in the treatment of the burnt skin tissue defects (Shanmugarajan et al., 2021). Another study indicates vitamin C with squalene bioconjugate promotes epidermal thickening and collagen production in human skin (Gref et al., 2020). The studies on squalene in animal models confirm the activity in Epidermal growth factor (EGF), act as scavenger and a source of energy in the membrane system (Kim, 1999).

POLYUNSATURATED HYDROCARBON

Squalene is a substance that acts as an intermediary in the metabolism of sterols and cholesterol, hence it can be found in both the tissues of mammals and plants. Six isoprene units combine to generate the polyunsaturated hydrocarbon squalene, which has the formula $C_{30}H_{50}$. The laboratory of Nobel Laureate Konrad Bloch was the first to propose that squalene cyclization to lanosterol is a step of cholesterol synthesis (Woodward & Bloch, 1953).

Figure 1. Chemical structure of squalene

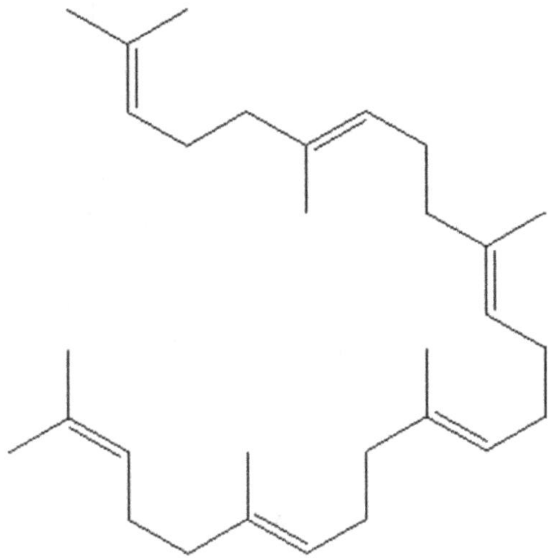

BIOACTIVE COMPOUNDS FROM PLANTS

Plants produced several useful bioactive compounds commonly known as secondary metabolites, having an important role in their growth and reproduction (Vanisree et al., 2004).

Hylocereus undatus

A study on flesh and the peel of the fruit of *Hylocereus undatus* using water and immediately vacuum-distilled for 5 h, yielding squalene (13.2%) as major constituents. The compounds were identified using gas chromatography-mass spectrometry. The biological test on the peel and crude flesh extract reveals active against 5-Lipoxygenase (81%) and AChE (>80%) respectively (Chester et al., 2017).). Another study confirms the wound healing potential of aqueous leaves, flower, and fruit plup of *Hylocereus undatus*. The results compare the wound healing activity between different parts of plant and found higher activity on the leaves and flower compared to fruit pulp.

Abroma augusta

Abroma augusta plant is indigenously used in the treatment of cuts, swellings, sores, and bruises. The fresh leaves of *Abroma augusta* were macerated with n-hexane and further purified with ethyl acetate and methanol fractions. The methanol fraction was purified and identified squalene from FT-IR, UV/Vis and GC-MS. The study indicates the anti-inflammatory activity on animal model (Latief et al., 2020).

Hemigraphis colorata

Hemigraphis colorata is traditional used as wound healing plant in many tribes in India. The dried leaves were subjected to Soxhlet extraction using n-hexane solvent. The study reveals the presence of squalene (Safna et al., 2020). The crude extract (i.e., aqueous and methanol) possess wound healing properties and were confirmed by many researchers using animal models (Subramoniam et al., 2001).

Prunus mume

The fruits of *Prunus mume* were underwent ethanol extraction. The extract was purified and fractionated by column chromatography. the purified subfractions contains squalene (Kim & Huh, 2021). There is no comprehensive report on the wound healing potential of *Prunus mume* but another species from Prunus genus (*Prunus spinosa)* from the fruits were found increased wound healing rates by promoting granulation tissue, epidermal regeneration, and angiogenesis (Ayla et al., 2017). There is a need of further phytochemical investigation on *Prunus spinosa* particularly squalene.

Clematis flammula

The aerial part of *Clematis flammula* (Ranunculaceae) has been traditionally used in the treatment of skin diseases including mycotic infection in the Tunisian traditional medicine. The plant contains squalene and triterpenoids such as anemonin. The study concluded with strong support for the effective wound healing activity of anemonin used as key ingredient in cream (Saidi et al., 2018).

Amarant Oil

Amaranth oil is extracted from the seeds of two species of the genus Amaranthus (*A. cruentus and A. hypochondriacus*). The study indicates its good wound healing potential in animal models as suggested to contain high content of squalene. The study assessed the thermal burn injury in animal model (Chulak et al., 2021). Some researcher found that Amaranth seed oil contain squalene as they fractionated in a bench-scale short-path distillation unit to obtain fractions rich in squalene (Sun et al., 1997).

Carica papaya

The aqueous extract of *Carica papaya* leaves strong suggest the wound healing activities in animal model (Mahmood et al., 2005). Moreover, a second study on fresh leaves of the plants were used for leaf juice extraction and were found active in cell-based assays. The results showed that the extract significantly protected skin fibroblasts from H_2O_2-induced oxidative stress in both pre-and post-treatment (Khor et al., 2021). The researcher proposed that the activity of leaf juice extract was due to the presence of rutin, a well-known flavonoid for its wound healing properties (Khor et al., 2021). However, squalene is also present in small percentage due to nature of extraction method. Therefore, we proposed the hypothesis that the skin protecting activity of the extract could be the synergistic effect of rutin and squalene.

Canthium coromandelicum

The methanolic extract from the leaves of *Canthium coromandelicum* contain abundant of squalene identified by GC-MS (Sasikala & Chandra Mohan, 2014). *Canthium coromandelicum* leaves possess the wound healing activity on animal

Figure 2. Some medicinal plants contain squalene

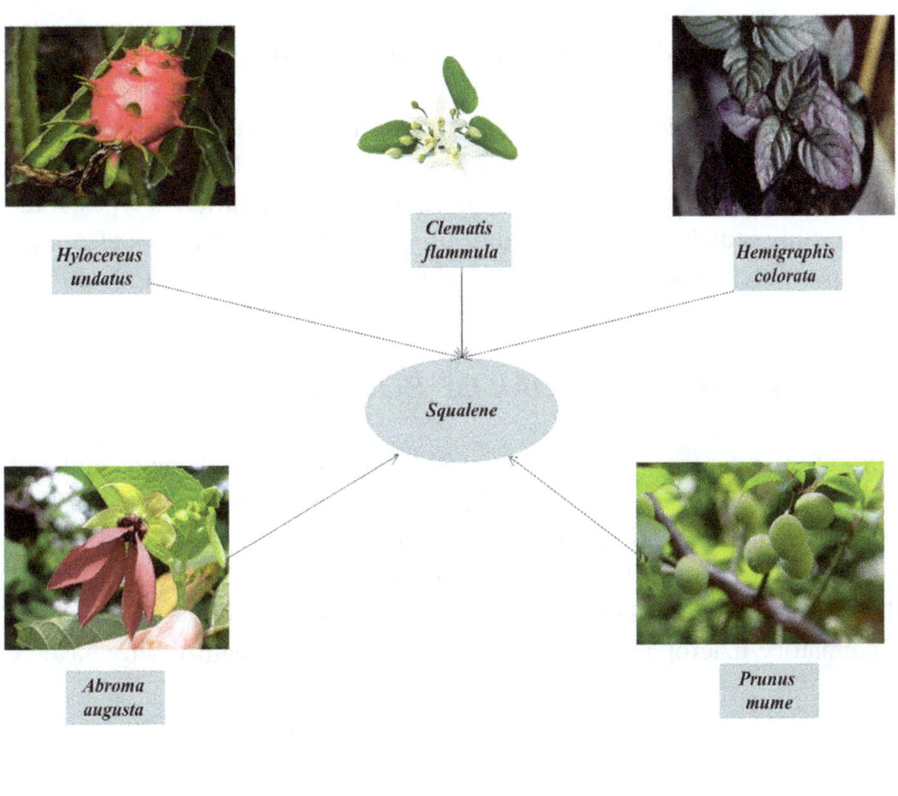

studies. The ethanolic extract was reported greater activity compared to cipladine (Mohan et al., 2014).

BIOACTIVE COMPOUNDS FROM ANIMAL SOURCE

Since ancient times, the inventory of therapeutic ingredients utilised in many cultures has included animals and products produced from their various organs (Lev, 2003). The most popular parenteral anticoagulants are heparins. The only type of heparin now utilized in the USA is obtained from swine, despite the fact that it can be extracted from a variety of animal sources (McCarthy et al., 2020).

Centrophorus squamosus (Shark Liver Oil)

Squalene and alkylglycerols are both present in shark liver oil, which is an old cure used by fishermen on Norway's and Sweden's west coasts. According to the folk medical tradition, giving shark liver oil in doses of 500 mg twice daily to elderly patients before surgery led to a considerable rise in WBC, lymphocytes, IgM, and IgA levels in the immediate aftermath of surgery (Palmieri et al., 2014). A second study indicate shark liver oil emulgel showed wound healing activity in burn wound model compared to standard formulations (Allahbaksh Auti et al., 2021).

Periplaneta americana (American Cockroach)

American cockroach is the key ingredient in traditional Chinese medicine commonly known as Kangfuxin in treating different kind of wounds, burn and ulcers. The ethanolic extract where purified and identified Squalene and different types of fatty acids. The study indicates good wound healing activity in animal model compare with total polysaccharides, total protein, and negative control (Zhu et al., 2018).

WOUND HEALING POTENTIAL OF SQUALENE

Squalene (SQ) possesses preventive effects against skin damage and anti-inflammatory properties. It is thought that the wound healing potential of SQ is due to its immunomodulation activity of macrophages. SQ induced an increase in the synthesis of anti-inflammatory cytokines, such as IL-10, IL-13, and IL-4, and a decrease in proinflammatory signals, such as TNF-α and NF-κB in M1 proinflammatory macrophages. The study was performed with macrophage cell line experimental model after SQ treatment in a human monocyte cell line (THP-1), which was differentiated into M1 macrophages (Sánchez-Quesada et al., 2018).

In 40 healthy female individuals (>50 years of age), SemoSqualene®, an oral supplement high in the polyunsaturated aliphatic hydrocarbon squalene was employed. For 90 days, a high dose of squalene (13.5–27 g per day) reduced face wrinkles, lowered skin responsiveness to UV, improved type I procollagen gene expression, and decreased UV induced DNA damage and apoptosis (Cho et al., 2009).

SQ was extracted from pumpkin seed oil to evaluate its potential against COVID-19 (Hataminia & Farhadian, 2017) and the microemulsion containing SQ with a concentration of 10 mg/ml was prepared using the titration method (Golmohammadzadeh et al., 2017). The treatment group received 5 mg of intravenous squalene twice a day and standard treatment for 6 days, while controls received only standard treatment. After 6 days of treatment, clinical and CT scan changes were evaluated and compared in intervention and control groups. The need for oxygen therapy ($p=0.020$), 2 days of no fever ($p=0.025$), cough alleviation ($p=0.010$), and lung high-resolution computed tomography improvement ($p=0.033$) were significantly different between cases and controls within 7 days of admission. No adverse effects were observed in the treatment group (Golmohammadzadeh et al., 2017).

There were several studies confirmed the pre-clinical activity of squalene or natural source containing squalene as wound healing agent on animal studies using wound model such as burn model (Shanmugarajan et al., 2021; Mohan et al., 2014). It is unfortunate that none of the given above studies were carry forward for clinical trials.

CONCLUSION

There are several bioactive compounds from natural sources that possess wound healing activities. The nature has gifted abundant of phytochemical compounds inside the natural sources. They are known as secondary metabolites. The wound healing activity of squalene works synergistically with other bioactivity compounds such as rutin, chitosan and oleic acid (Asfour et al., 2017). There is a need to standardize the bioactive metabolites in medicinal plants by controlling and monitoring each parameter such as plant stress, growth, collection, drying and extraction factors. The optimization of factors will be able to determine the quality of medicinal plants and their bioactivities. Moreover, there is a need to develop more robust methodologies for quick standardization technique using advance artificial intelligence and machine learning approach to confirms the potential bioactive compounds.

ACKNOWLEDGMENT

MSA, YJK and QL acknowledge the support from Xiamen University Malaysia.

REFERENCES

Abuobeid, R., Sánchez-Marco, J., Felices, M. J., Arnal, C., Burillo, J. C., Lasheras, R., Busto, R., Lasunción, M. A., Rodríguez-Yoldi, M. J., Martínez-Beamonte, R., & Osada, J. (2022, April). Squalene through Its Post-Squalene Metabolites Is a Modulator of Hepatic Transcriptome in Rabbits. *International Journal of Molecular Sciences*, *23*(8), 4172. doi:10.3390/ijms23084172 PMID:35456988

Akin, G., Arslan, F. N., Karuk Elmasa, S. N., & Yilmaz, I. (2018, March). Cold-pressed pumpkin seed (<em>Cucurbita pepo</em> L.) oils from the central Anatolia region of Turkey: Characterization of phytosterols, squalene, tocols, phenolic acids, carotenoids and fatty acid bioactive compounds. *Grasas y Aceites*, *69*(1), 232. doi:10.3989/gya.0668171

Allahbaksh Auti, S., Kumar Jat, R., Das, S. K., & Shukla, S. S. T. (2021, July). Determination of Wound Healing Activity of Shark Liver Oil using Burn Wound Model in Wistar Rats. *Journal of Young Pharmacists: JYP*, *13*(2), 113–117. doi:10.5530/jyp.2021.13.24

Angeletti, L. R., Agrimi, U., French, D., Curia, C., & Mariani-Costantini, R. (1992, July). L. Angeletti, U. Agrimi, D. French, C. Curia, and R. Mariani-Costantini, "Healing rituals and sacred serpents. *Lancet*, *340*(8813), 223–225. doi:10.1016/0140-6736(92)90480-Q PMID:1353146

Asfour, M. H., Elmotasem, H., Mostafa, D. M., & Salama, A. A. A. (2017, December). Chitosan based Pickering emulsion as a promising approach for topical application of rutin in a solubilized form intended for wound healing: In vitro and in vivo study. *International Journal of Pharmaceutics*, *534*(1–2), 325–338. doi:10.1016/j.ijpharm.2017.10.044 PMID:29074391

Ayla, Ş., Günal, M. Y., Sayın Şakul, A. A., Biçeroğlu, Ö., Özdemir, E. M., Okur, M. E., Polat, D. Ç., Üstündağ Okur, N., & Bilgiç, B. E. (2017). Effects of Prunus spinosa L. fruits on experimental wound healing. *Medeni. Med. J.*, *32*(3), 152–158. doi:10.5222/MMJ.2017.152

Catchpole, O. J., von Kamp, J.-C., & Grey, J. B. (1997, October). Extraction of Squalene from Shark Liver Oil in a Packed Column Using Supercritical Carbon Dioxide. *Industrial & Engineering Chemistry Research*, *36*(10), 4318–4324. doi:10.1021/ie9702237

Chester, K., Zahiruddin, S., Ahmad, A., Khan, W., Paliwal, S., & Ahmad, S. (2017). *Bioautography-based Identification of Antioxidant Metabolites of Solanum nigrum L. and Exploration Its Hepatoprotective Potential*. Academic Press.

Cho, S., Choi, C.-W., Lee, D. H., Won, C.-H., Kim, S. M., Lee, S., Lee, M.-J., & Chung, J. H. (2009, June). High-dose squalene ingestion increases type I procollagen and decreases ultraviolet-induced DNA damage in human skin in vivo but is associated with transient adverse effects. *Clinical and Experimental Dermatology*, *34*(4), 500–508. doi:10.1111/j.1365-2230.2008.03133.x PMID:19522983

Chulak, O. L., Gozhenko, A. I., Chulak, Y. L., Chulak, L. D., & Badiuk, N. S. (2021). Morphology of thermal burn injury under the use of amarant oil (amaránthus). *Pharmacologyonline*, *1*, 1–5.

Couvreur, P., & Vauthier, C. (2006, July). Nanotechnology: Intelligent Design to Treat Complex Disease. *Pharmaceutical Research*, *23*(7), 1417–1450. doi:10.100711095-006-0284-8 PMID:16779701

Golmohammadzadeh, S., Farhadian, N., Biriaee, A., Dehghani, F., & Khameneh, B. (2017, October). Preparation, characterization and in vitro evaluation of microemulsion of raloxifene hydrochloride. *Drug Development and Industrial Pharmacy*, *43*(10), 1619–1625. doi:10.1080/03639045.2017.1328430 PMID:28489426

Gref, R., Deloménie, C., Maksimenko, A., Gouadon, E., Percoco, G., Lati, E., Desmaële, D., Zouhiri, F., & Couvreur, P. (2020, December). Vitamin C–squalene bioconjugate promotes epidermal thickening and collagen production in human skin. *Scientific Reports*, *10*(1), 16883. doi:10.103841598-020-72704-1 PMID:33037252

Hataminia, F., & Farhadian, N. (2017, September). A novel experimental method for adsorption of fatty acids from pumpkin seed oil in the presence of iron oxide nanoparticles: Experimental and SA – LOOCV – GRBF mathematical modeling. *Colloids and Surfaces. A, Physicochemical and Engineering Aspects*, *528*, 30–40. doi:10.1016/j.colsurfa.2017.05.042

Hataminia, F., Farhadian, N., Karimi, M., & Ebrahimi, M. (2018, October). A novel method for squalene extraction from pumpkin seed oil using magnetic nanoparticles and exploring the inhibition effect of extracted squalene on angiogenesis property. *Journal of the Taiwan Institute of Chemical Engineers*, *91*, 1–9. doi:10.1016/j.jtice.2018.05.017

He, H.-P., Corke, H., & Cai, J.-G. (2003, December). Supercritical Carbon Dioxide Extraction of Oil and Squalene from Amaranthus Grain. *Journal of Agricultural and Food Chemistry*, *51*(27), 7921–7925. doi:10.1021/jf030488y PMID:14690374

Khor, B. K. K., Chear, N. J. Y., Azizi, J., & Khaw, K. Y. (2021). Chemical composition, antioxidant and cytoprotective potentials of carica papaya leaf extracts: A comparison of supercritical fluid and conventional extraction methods. *Molecules (Basel, Switzerland)*, *26*(5), 1489. Advance online publication. doi:10.3390/molecules26051489 PMID:33803330

Kim, J. S. (1999). Healing effects of Squalene on the epidermis in Burned Mouse. *Korean J. Electron Microsocpy*, *29*(2), 163–175.

Kim, S.-K., & Karadeniz, F. (2012). Biological Importance and Applications of Squalene and Squalane. Advances in Food and Nutrition Research, 65. doi:10.1016/B978-0-12-416003-3.00014-7

Kim, S. M., & Huh, C. K. (2021, October). Isolation and identification of squalene as an antioxidative compound from the fruits of Prunus mume. *Journal of Food Processing and Preservation*, *45*(10), 1–10. doi:10.1111/jfpp.15810

Latief, M., Muhaimin, M., Amanda, H., Prahandika, G., & Tarigan, I. L. (2020, December). "Anti-inflammatory activities of squalene compound of methanol extract of Abroma augusta L," *J. Teknol. Lab.*, *9*(2), 176–185. doi:10.29238/teknolabjournal.v9i2.228

Lev, E. (2003, March). Traditional healing with animals (zootherapy): Medieval to present-day Levantine practice. *Journal of Ethnopharmacology*, *85*(1), 107–118. doi:10.1016/S0378-8741(02)00377-X PMID:12576209

Lozano-Grande, M. A., Dávila-Ortiz, G., García-Dávila, J., Ríos-Cortés, G., Espitia-Rangel, E., & Martínez-Ayala, A. L. (2019, October). Optimisation of Microwave-Assisted Extraction of Squalene from A maranthus spp. Seeds. *The Journal of Microwave Power and Electromagnetic Energy*, *53*(4), 243–258. doi:10.1080/08327823.2019.1677429

Mahmood, A. A., Sidik, K., & Salmah, I. (2005). Wound Healing Activity of Carica papaya L. Aqueous Leaf Extract in Rats. *International Journal of Molecular Medicine and Advanced Sciences*, *1*(4), 398–401.

McCarthy, C. P., Vaduganathan, M., Solomon, E., Sakhuja, R., Piazza, G., Bhatt, D. L., Connors, J. M., & Patel, N. K. (2020, February). Running thin: Implications of a heparin shortage. *Lancet*, *395*(10223), 534–536. doi:10.1016/S0140-6736(19)33135-6 PMID:31982034

Mohan, S. C., Sasikala, K., & Anand, T. (2014). Antimicrobial and Wound Healing Potential of Canthium coromandelicum Leaf Extract-A Preliminary Study. *Research Journal of Phytochemistry*, *8*(2), 35–41. doi:10.3923/rjphyto.2014.35.41

Ortega, J., Martínez Zavala, A., Hernández, M., & Díaz Reyes, J. (2012, December). Analysis of trans fatty acids production and squalene variation during amaranth oil extraction. *Open Chemistry*, *10*(6), 1773–1778. doi:10.247811532-012-0104-4

Owen, R. W., Haubner, R., Würtele, G., Hull, W. E., Spiegelhalder, B., & Bartsch, H. (2004, August). Olives and olive oil in cancer prevention. *European Journal of Cancer Prevention*, *13*(4), 319–326. doi:10.1097/01.cej.0000130221.19480.7e PMID:15554560

Palmieri, B., Pennelli, A., & Di Cerbo, A. (2014, December). Jurassic surgery and immunity enhancement by alkyglycerols of shark liver oil. *Lipids in Health and Disease*, *13*(1), 178. doi:10.1186/1476-511X-13-178 PMID:25427577

Perez, R. M., Vargas, R., & Ortiz, Y. D. (2005, August). Wound healing properties of Hylocereus undatus on diabetic rats. *Phytotherapy Research*, *19*(8), 665–668. doi:10.1002/ptr.1724 PMID:16177967

Prakashbabu, B. C., Vijay, D., George, S., Kodiyil, S., Nair, S. N., Gopalan, A. K., Juliet, S., & Ravindran, R. (2017, August). Wound Healing and Anti-Inflammatory Activity of Methanolic Extract of Gmelina arborea and Hemigraphis colorata in Rats. *International Journal of Current Microbiology and Applied Sciences*, *6*(8), 3116–3122. doi:10.20546/ijcmas.2017.608.373

Riaz, H., Raza, S., Aslam, M., Ahmad, M., Ahmad, M., & Maria, P. (2018, March). An Updated Review of Pharmacological, Standardization Methods and Formulation Development of Rutin. *Journal of Pure & Applied Microbiology*, *12*(1), 127–132. doi:10.22207/JPAM.12.1.16

Rosales-Garcia, T., Jimenez-Martinez, C., & Davila-Ortiz, G. (2017). Squalene Extraction: Biological Sources and Extraction Methods. *Int. J. Environ. Agric. Biotechnol.*, *2*(4), 1662–1670. doi:10.22161/ijeab/2.4.26

Rotondo, A., Salvo, A., Gallo, V., Rastrelli, L., & Dugo, G. (2017, November). Quick unreferenced NMR quantification of Squalene in vegetable oils. *European Journal of Lipid Science and Technology*, *119*(11), 1700151. doi:10.1002/ejlt.201700151

Sabeenafarvin, K., Anandan, R., Senthilkumar, S., Shiny, K., Sankar, T., & Thankappan, T. (2004, September). Effect of squalene on tissue defense system in isoproterenol-induced myocardial infarction in rats. *Pharmacological Research*, *50*(3), 231–236. doi:10.1016/j.phrs.2004.03.004 PMID:15225664

Safna, M. I., Visakh, U. V., & Gangadharan, A. (2020). Biological activity of hexane extract of Hemigraphis colorata, an indigenous wound healing plant. *Materials Today: Proceedings*, *25*, 294–297. doi:10.1016/j.matpr.2020.01.461

Saidi, R., Ghrab, F., Kallel, R., Feki, A. E., Boudawara, T., Chesné, C., Ammar, E., & Jarraya, R. M. (2018). Tunisian *Clematis flammula* Essential Oil Enhances Wound Healing: GC-MS Analysis, Biochemical and Histological Assessment. *Journal of Oleo Science*, *67*(11), 1483–1499. doi:10.5650/jos.ess18056 PMID:30404969

Sánchez-Quesada, C., López-Biedma, A., Toledo, E., & Gaforio, J. J. (2018, September). Squalene Stimulates a Key Innate Immune Cell to Foster Wound Healing and Tissue Repair. *Evidence-Based Complement. Altern. Med*, *1*, 1–9. doi:10.1155/2018/9473094 PMID:30363968

Sasikala, K., & Chandra Mohan, S. (2014). Total phenolic, Flavanoid contents and GC-MS analysis of canthium coromandelicum leaves extract. *International Journal of Pharmacy and Pharmaceutical Sciences*, *6*(8), 379–381.

Shanmugarajan, T. S., Selvan, N. K., & Uppuluri, V. N. V. A. (2021, December). Development and Characterization of Squalene-Loaded Topical Agar-Based Emulgel Scaffold: Wound Healing Potential in Full-Thickness Burn Model. *The International Journal of Lower Extremity Wounds*, *20*(4), 364–373. doi:10.1177/1534734620921629 PMID:32502363

Spanova, M., & Daum, G. (2011, November). Squalene – biochemistry, molecular biology, process biotechnology, and applications. *European Journal of Lipid Science and Technology*, *113*(11), 1299–1320. doi:10.1002/ejlt.201100203

Srinivasaiah, N., Dugdall, H., Barrett, S., & Drew, P. (2007, October). A point prevalence survey of wounds in north-east England. *Journal of Wound Care*, *16*(10), 413–419. doi:10.12968/jowc.2007.16.10.27910 PMID:18065016

Subramoniam, A., Evans, D. A., Rajasekharan, S., & Sreekandan Nair, G. (2001). Effect of Hemigraphis colorata (Blume) H. G. Hallier leaf on wound healing and inflammation in mice. *Indian Journal of Pharmacology*, *33*(4), 283–285.

Sun, H., Wiesenborn, D., Tostenson, K., Gillespie, J., & Rayas-Duarte, P. (1997). Fractionation of squalene from amaranth seed oil. *J. Am. Oil Chem. Soc.*, *74*(4), 413–418. . doi:10.1007/s11746-997-0099-8

Vanisree, M., Lee, C.-Y., Lo, S.-F., Nalawade, S. M., Lin, C. Y., & Tsay, H.-S. (2004). Studies on the production of some important secondary metabolites from medicinal plants by plant tissue cultures. *Botanical Bulletin of Academia Sinica*, *45*, 1–22.

Woodward, R. B., & Bloch, K. (1953, April). The cyclization of squalene in cholesterol synthesis. *Journal of the American Chemical Society*, *75*(8), 2023–2024. doi:10.1021/ja01104a535

Xiao, S., Zhang, Y., Xie, J., & Wen, Z. (2018, December). Ultrasonic-assisted extraction of squalene and vitamin E based oil from Zizyphi Spinosae Semen and evaluation of its antioxidant activity. *Journal of Food Measurement and Characterization*, *12*(4), 2844–2854. doi:10.100711694-018-9899-9

Zhu, J.-J., Yao, S., Guo, X., Yue, B.-S., Ma, X.-Y., & Li, J. (2018, January). Bioactivity-Guided Screening of Wound-Healing Active Constituents from American Cockroach (Periplaneta americana). *Molecules (Basel, Switzerland)*, *23*(1), 101. doi:10.3390/molecules23010101 PMID:29361715

Chapter 5
Educating Pharmacology to T&CM Students Using Mnemonics

Muhammad Shahzad Aslam
https://orcid.org/0000-0003-2728-6726
School of Traditional Chinese Medicine, Xiamen University Malaysia, Malaysia

EXECUTIVE SUMMARY

The scientific field of pharmacology aims to give a thorough understanding of how medications affect the human body. In Malaysia, the bachelor's degree programme of traditional Malay medicine, traditional Chinese medicine, acupuncture, Moxibustion and Tuina, Siddha medicine, homeopathy, chiropractic, and osteopathy contain two credit hours for the subject pharmacology. The student faces a time challenge to understand the broad concept of pharmacology and memorising some important drugs classification. Therefore, using mnemonic is an interesting method to develop and understanding and memorising drug classifications.

INTRODUCTION

Traditional and complementary medicine (T&CM) dates back to ancient times. It has changed to reflect many philosophical perspectives and cultural antecedents. The fusion of T&CM and Western medicine is still in its infancy in Malaysia. In Kepala Batas, Pulau Pinang, the first integrated hospital was founded in 2007. It offers cancer patients acupuncture, Malay massage, and herbal therapy. T&CM education in Malaysia has for 50 years been following China's traditional Chinese medicine education curriculums. Currently, the Division of T&CM, Ministry of Health, and

DOI: 10.4018/978-1-6684-7828-8.ch005

Ministry of Higher Education has approved 11 institutions to offer T&CM education. Students may major in Chinese herbal medicine (traditional Chinese medicine), acupuncture, or other T&CM clinical subjects, such as Tui-na, natural medicine, homeopathy, Malay medicine, Malay massage, ayurveda medicine, chiropractic, reflexology, aromatherapy, and Islamic medicine (Kim, 2017).

SUFFIXES IN DRUG MNEMONICS

The inclusion of prefixes and suffixes are common in medical terminology. The easiest way to memories the drugs name is understanding the presence of prefix and suffix in a drug name. A prefix is a letter or group of letters, which is added to the beginning of a word in order to form a different word whereas a morpheme added at the end of a word to form a derivative is termed as suffix. The suffix use in β-adrenceptor antagonist drugs (proprano**lol**, nado**lol**, timo**lol**, metopro**lol**, ateno**lol**, betaxo**lol**, nebivo**lol**, pindo**lol**, acebuto**lol**, carteo**lol**, carvedi**lol**) consist of ***"-lol"***. The suffux use in α-adrenceptor antagonist drugs (prazo**sin**, doxazo**sin**, terazo**sin**, tamsulo**sin**) consist of ***"-sin"***. The drugs used in the treatment of hypertension consist of various class of drugs such as diuretics, α-blocker, β-blocker, vasodilators, angiotensin-converting enzyme (ace) inhibitors and angiotensin receptor blockers. To memorise the vasodilators drugs (nife**dipine**, amlo**dipine**) consist of ***"-dipine".*** Nifedipine and amlodipine categorize under calcium channel blocker (Russell, 1988). The suffix for thiazide diuretics (hydrochloro**thiazide**) is ***"-thiazide"***. Spironol**actone** and ald**actone** are potassium sparing diuretic that contain suffix ***"-actone"***. Vasopressin antagonists (coni**vaptan**, tol**vaptan**) reduces water reabsorption, increases plasma sodium concentration and vasodilation contain suffix ***"-vaptan"*** (Schrier, 2006). Angiotensin-II-receptor antagonists (val**sartan**. cande**sartan**, irbe**sartan**, lo**sartan**, olme**sartan**) also known as sartans contains suffix as ***"-sartans"***. ACE inhibitors such as capto**pril**, lisino**pril** reduce blood pressure by dilating blood vessels, thus reducing the heart's workload (Beaulieu et al., 1993). It contains ***"-pril"*** as suffix. Flecai**nide** and encai**nide**, belong to class IC antiarrhythmic drugs contain suffix ***"-nide"***. Dofeti**lide** and Ibuti**lide** are class III antiarrhythmic drugs that work by blocking potassium channels contains suffix***"-lide"***. Cholesterol-lowering drugs (atorva**statin**, simva**statin**) are famous with another name called statins because of the suffix ***"-statin"***. Histamine H2-receptor antagonists (H2-blockers) are used to treat duodenal ulcers (Spiro, 1983). They are used to treat gastric ulcers and for some conditions, such as Zollinger-Ellison disease, in which the stomach produces too much acid. The well-know suffix used to memorize the drugs (cime**tidine**, famo**tidine**, niza**tidine**, rani**tidine**) contain ***"-tidine"***. Frova**triptan** and ele**triptan** are common serotonin agonist used in the treatment of used to treat the symptoms of migraine headache. Renin inhibitors (enal**kiren**, alis**kiren**, remi**kiren**) prevents catalytic activity of renin that results in arteriolar dilation, decreased aldosterone secretion, increased sodium and water excretion (Allikmets, 2007). It contains ***"-kiren"*** as suffix. Natriuretic peptides contain suffix ***"-tide"*** (nesiri**tide**, carperi**tide**) are agonists of natriuretic peptide receptors that are clinically used in heart failure (Chen & Burnett, 1999). Vasopeptidase inhibitors (omapa**trilat**, fasido**trilat,** sampa**trilat**) are responsible for decreases metabolism of natriuretic peptides and formation of angiotensin II (Sarzani et al., 2008). The drug include under the following category contains the suffix ***"-trilat"***. Endothelin antagonists are nonselective antagonists of endothelin ETA and ETB receptors that produce vasodialation (Verhaar et al., 1998). Bos**entan**, maci**tentan** are examples under the following category used in the treatment of pulmonary arterial hypertension (Bedan et al., 2018). It contains suffix as a ***"-entan"***. Calcitonin gene-related peptide antagonists are antagonists of the calcitonin gene-related peptide (CGRP) receptor that block some central and peripheral (vasodilator) actions of Calcitonin gene-related peptide (CGRP) (Miranda et al., 2013). It is indicated in the treatment of migrane. Telca**gepant** and olce**gepant** are drugs used as CGRP and contains suffix ***"-gepant"***. Corticisteroids (flutica**sone**, predni**sone**) are responsible to reduce the inflammation (Belda et al., 2007) and the suffix that come at the end is ***"-sone"***. Methylxanthines (theo**phylline**, and dy**phylline**) are known as bronchodilators, cardiac stimulators, increased skeletal muscle strength (diaphragm) and used in the treatment of asthma and coronary obstructive pulmonary disease (COPD)(Katzung, 2015). ***"-phylline"*** is the suffix used under methyxanthines category. Leukotriene antagonists (monte**lukast**, zafir**lukast**) block airway response to exercise and antigen challenge (Busse et al., 1999). They are responsible to Block leukotriene D4 receptors and indicated in the prophylaxis of asthma, especially in children and in aspirin-induced asthma. The suffix given under the category is ***"-lukast"***. Anti-interleukin-5 pathway antibodies, miscellaneous antibodies (Mepoliz**umab**, Dupil**umab**) and IgE antibody (Omaliz**umab**) are indicated to reduces frequency of asthma exacerbations and ***"-umab"*** as suffix used. Benzodiazepines are clinically used in acute anxiety states, panic attacks, generalized anxiety, disorder, insomnia, sleep disorders, relaxation of skeletal muscle, anesthesia and seizure disorders (Longo & Johnson, 2000). They bind to specific GABAA receptor subunits at central nervous system (CNS) neuronal synapses facilitating GABA-mediated chloride ion channel opening frequency and enhance membrane.

There are two common suffixes used ***"-zepam"*** and ***"-zolam"***. Some common benzodiazepines include alpra**zolam**, esta**zolam**, mida**zolam**, tria**zolam** clona**zepam**, dia**zepam**, flura**zepam**, lora**zepam**, oxa**zepam**, qua**zepam**, and tema**zepam**. Barbiturates have a dose-dependent depressant effects on the CNS including sedation and relief of anxiety, amnesia, hypnosis, anesthesia, coma and respiratory depression. Amo**barbital**, buta**barbital**, mepho**barbital**, pento**barbital**, pheno**barbital** and seco**barbital** are common drugs under bartiburates and the suffix ***"-barbital"*** has been named. Gabapentinoids (pre**gabalin**, miro**gabalin**) are clinically indicated in focal seizures, neuropathic pain, postherpetic neuralgia and anxiety. ***"-gabalin"*** is used as suffix in list of gabapentinoids drugs. Drugs used for local anesthesia have classified into amides and esters. The common suffix used in amides and esters are ***"-caine"*** such as lido**caine**, Bupiva**caine**, Chloropro**caine** and Co**caine**. The following drugs blockade the sodium channels, as a result slows, then blocks, action potential propagation. Carbidopa and levodopa combination is used to treat Parkinson's disease contains suffix as ***"-dopa"***. The COMT inhibitors, tolca**pone** and entaca**pone**, are a new class of Parkinson's medications contains the suffix as ***"-pone"***. The drugs inhibit COMT (catechol-O-methyltransferase) in periphery and does not enter CNS. Antimuscarinic agents are the predominant pharmacological treatment for patients with overactive bladder (OAB) (Kay et al., 2005b). These drugs are thought to act primarily through antagonism at muscarinic M3 receptors located at neuromuscular junctions in the human bladder detrusor muscle. Dari**fenacin** and Soli**fenac** are commonly used in OAB that contain the suffix ***"-fenac"*** (Kay et al., 2005a). Some antimuscarinic agent has used in the treatment of Parkinson disease such as Benz**tropine** to reduce the tremor and rigidity, whereas a**tropi**ne (treatment of poisoning by susceptible organophosphorus nerve agents) and **tropi**camide (mydriasis and cycloplegia in diagnostic procedures) were belong to similar category. The prefix and suffix used are **"-tropi"**. Second-generation antipsychotics have clinically indicated in schizophrenia, bipolar disorder and major depression. Aripiprazole, brexpiprazole, clozapine, olanzapine, risperidone and ziprasidone are the common example and consist of suffix such as ***"-azole"***, **"-zapine"** and, ***"-done"***. Opioid agonists such as methadone and hydrocodone contain suffix ***"-done"***. Opioid receptor (nalo**xone**, naltre**xone**) antagonist has commonly used in the treatment of opioid overdose, opioid addiction and alcoholism (Wang, 2019). The suffix consists of **"-xone"**. Vitamin B12 such as cyanocobalamin and hydroxocobalamin contain suffix ***"-cobalamin"***. Statins such as atorvastatin, simvastatin, rosuvastatin, and pitavastatin contain suffix ***"-statin"*** inhibit HMG-CoA reductase and clinically indicated in atherosclerotic vascular disease (primary and secondary prevention) and acute coronary syndromes. Meglitinide analogs are insulin secretagogue that are similar to sulfonylureas with some overlap in binding sites and is used in the treatment of type-2 diabetes. Repa**glinide**, nate**glinide** and miti**glinide** are some common examples and consist of suffix ***"-glinide"***. Dipeptidyl peptidase-4 (dpp-4) inhibitors are type-2 diabetic drugs that reduces post-meal glucose excursions, increases glucose-mediated insulin release, lowers glucagon levels, slows gastric emptying, and decreases appetite. Sita**gliptin**, saxa**gliptin**, lina**gliptin**, alo**gliptin**, and vilda**gliptin** are common drugs and contain the suffix ***"-gliptin"***. Sodium-glucose co-transporter 2 (sglt2) inhibitors (Cana**gliflozin**, dapa**gliflozin**, and empa**gliflozin**) contain suffix ***"-gliflozin"*** and block renal glucose resorption and indicated in type-2 diabetes. Penicillins are clinically indicated to treat streptococcal infections, meningococcal infections and neurosyphilis. They prevent bacterial cell wall synthesis by binding to and inhibiting cell wall transpeptidases. Peni**cillin** G, peni**cillin** V, benzathine peni**cillin**, naf**cillin**, oxa**cillin**, ampi**cillin**, amoxi**cillin**, pipera**cillin.** The common suffix ***"-cillin"*** is present in drugs under the following category. Carbapenems is indicated in pneumonia and sepsis. It prevents bacterial cell wall synthesis by binding to and inhibiting cell wall transpeptidases. Imipenem, meropenem, doripenem, and ertapenem are common examples and contain suffix "*-penem*". Monobactams (Aztreo**nam**, tigemo**nam**) are indicated in infections caused by aerobic, gram-negative bacteria in patients with immediate hypersensitivity to penicillins. Glycopeptide is used in the infections caused by gram-positive bacteria including sepsis, endocarditis, and meningitis. It inhibits the cell wall synthesis by binding to the d-Ala-d-Ala terminus of nascent peptidoglycan. Dalba**vancin**, orita**vancin** and tela**vancin** are examples under the following category and contain the suffix **"-vancin"**. Macrolides (Erythro**mycin**, clatri**mycin**, azithro**mycin**) and lincosamide (clinda**mycin**) are having the bacteriostatic activity against susceptible bacteria and contain the suffix ***"-mycin"***. Streptogramins such as quinu**pristin** and dalfo**pristin** is indicated in infections caused by staphylococci or vancomycin resistant strains of E faecium. Aminoglycosides & spectinomycin contain similar suffix as macrolides and linocosamide. Fluoroquinolones (Cipro**floxacin**, levo**floxacin**, moxi**floxacin**, gemi**floxacin**) is indicated in the treatment of urinary tract infection, gastroenteritis, osteomyelitis and, anthrax (Majalekar & Shirote, 2020). The suffix observed in the following category is ***"-floxacin"***. Ketoconazole and Itraconazole are anti-fungal drugs and ***"-zole"*** as suffix present in the following drugs (Katzung, 2015; Brunton et al., 2011).

CONCLUSION

The biggest challenge that T&CM student in Malaysia faces to memorise the name of drugs. The number of credit hours for the subject pharmacology under Malaysian programme standards: traditional and complementary medicine, second Edition is only two hours (MQA, 2021) which gave lack of time. The current chapter will help student to memorise drugs names quickly.

REFERENCES

Allikmets, K. (2007). Aliskiren--An orally active renin inhibitor. Review of pharmacology, pharmacodynamics, kinetics, and clinical potential in the treatment of hypertension. *Vascular Health and Risk Management, 3*(6), 809–815.

Beaulieu, M., Nadeau, A., Lacourcière, Y., & Cléroux, J. (1993). Post-exercise reduction in blood pressure in hypertensive subjects: Effects of angiotensin converting enzyme inhibition. *British Journal of Clinical Pharmacology, 36*(4), 331–338. doi:10.1111/j.1365-2125.1993.tb00372.x PMID:12959311

Bedan, M., Grimm, D., Wehland, M., Simonsen, U., Infanger, M., & Krüger, M. (2018). A Focus on Macitentan in the Treatment of Pulmonary Arterial Hypertension. *Basic & Clinical Pharmacology & Toxicology, 123*(2), 103–113. doi:10.1111/bcpt.13033 PMID:29719121

Belda, J., Margarit, G., Martinez, C., Bellido-Casado, J., Casan, P., Torrejon, M., Brufal, M., Rodriguez-Jerez, F., & Sanchis, J. (2007). Anti-inflammatory effects of high-dose inhaled fluticasone versus oral prednisone in asthma exacerbations. *The European Respiratory Journal, 30*(6), 1143–1149. doi:10.1183/09031936.00050306 PMID:17690122

Brunton, L. L., Chabner, B. A., & Knollmann, B. C. (2011). The Pharmacological basis of Therapeutics. In L. L. Brunton, B. A. Chabner, & B. C. Knollmann (Eds.), *The pharmacological basis of Therapeutics*. Elsevier. https://linkinghub.elsevier.com/retrieve/pii/B97803234811060 00302

Busse, W. W., Mcgill, K. A., & Horwitz, R. J. (1999). Leukotriene pathway inhibitors in asthma and chronic obstructive pulmonary disease. *Clinical and Experimental Allergy, 29*(2), 110–115. doi:10.1046/j.1365-2222.1999.00019.x PMID:10421833

Chen, H. H., & Burnett, J. C. Jr. (1999). The Natriuretic Peptides in Heart Failure: Diagnostic and Therapeutic Potentials. *Proceedings of the Association of American Physicians, 111*(5), 406–416. doi:10.1111/paa.1999.111.5.406 PMID:10519161

Katzung, B. G. (2015). Basic & Clinical Pharmacology (14th ed.). McGraw Hill.

Kay, G. G., Abou-Donia, M. B., Messer, W. S. Jr, Murphy, D. G., Tsao, J. W., & Ouslander, J. G. (2005). Antimuscarinic Drugs for Overactive Bladder and Their Potential Effects on Cognitive Function in Older Patients. *Journal of the American Geriatrics Society, 53*(12), 2195–2201. doi:10.1111/j.1532-5415.2005.00537.x PMID:16398909

Kim, Y. J. (2017). The Current Studies of Education for a Traditional and Complementary Medicine in Malaysia. *Journal of Evidence-Based Complementary & Alternative Medicine*, *22*(4), 531–537. doi:10.1177/2156587217726882 PMID:28853309

Longo, L. P., & Johnson, B. (2000). Addiction: Part I. Benzodiazepines—Side Effects, Abuse Risk and Alternatives. *American Family Physician, 61*(7), 2121–2128. https://www.aafp.org/pubs/afp/issues/2000/0401/p2121.html

Majalekar, P. P., & Shirote, P. J. (2020). Fluoroquinolones: Blessings Or Curses. *Current Drug Targets*, *21*(13), 1354–1370. doi:10.2174/1389450121666200621193355 PMID:32564750

Miranda, L. P., Shi, L., Holder, J. R., Wright, M., Gegg, C. V., Johnson, E., Wild, K., Stenkilsson, M., Doellgast, G., Manning, B. H., & Salyers, K. (2013). Peptide antagonists of the calcitonin gene-related peptide (CGRP) receptor with improved pharmacokinetics and pharmacodynamics. *Biopolymers*, *100*(4), 422–430. doi:10.1002/bip.22270 PMID:23868210

MQA. (2021). *Program Standards: Traditional and Complementary Medicine*. PT Online. https://www.ptonline.com/articles/how-to-get-better-mfi-results

Russell, R. P. (1988). Side effects of calcium channel blockers. *Hypertension*, *11*(3_pt_2). doi:10.1161/01.HYP.11.3_Pt_2.II42 PMID:3280492

Sarzani, R., Salvi, F., Dessì-Fulgheri, P., & Rappelli, A. (2008). Renin–angiotensin system, natriuretic peptides, obesity, metabolic syndrome, and hypertension: An integrated view in humans. *Journal of Hypertension*, *26*(5), 831–843. doi:10.1097/HJH.0b013e3282f624a0 PMID:18398321

Schrier, R. W. (2006). Water and Sodium Retention in Edematous Disorders: Role of Vasopressin and Aldosterone. *The American Journal of Medicine*, *119*(7), S47–S53. doi:10.1016/j.amjmed.2006.05.007 PMID:16843085

Spiro, H. M. (1983). H2-blockers. *Journal of Clinical Gastroenterology*, *5*, 143–148. doi:10.1097/00004836-198312001-00014 PMID:6140282

Verhaar, M. C., Strachan, F. E., Newby, D. E., Cruden, N. L., Koomans, H. A., Rabelink, T. J., & Webb, D. J. (1998). Endothelin-A Receptor Antagonist–Mediated Vasodilatation Is Attenuated by Inhibition of Nitric Oxide Synthesis and by Endothelin-B Receptor Blockade. *Circulation*, *97*(8), 752–756. doi:10.1161/01.CIR.97.8.752 PMID:9498538

Wang, S. (2019). Historical Review: Opiate Addiction and Opioid Receptors. *Cell Transplantation*, *28*(3), 233–238. doi:10.1177/0963689718811060 PMID:30419763

Chapter 6
Enhancing Memory Using Mnemonics Acronym:
An Undergraduate Traditional Chinese Medicine Pharmacology Course

Muhammad Shahzad Aslam
https://orcid.org/0000-0003-2728-6726
School of Traditional Chinese Medicine, Xiamen University Malaysia, Malaysia

Dulmaa Lkhagvasuren
Independent Researcher, Mongolia

EXECUTIVE SUMMARY

Traditional Chinese medicine students find pharmacology challenging because it is complicated, yet they still need to understand facts about the mechanism of actions of drugs and how to use this knowledge in clinical settings. Mnemonics are strategies that can enhance learning and memory of course material. Mnemonics are memory techniques that aid in chunking and organising material to be learnt; as a result, they improve encoding and ease retrieval. There are variety of forms that include acronyms and acrostics (also known as first-letter mnemonics), the loci method, the pegword method, the keyword approach, auditory, visual, and kinesthetic mnemonics, and a group of semantic-based mnemonic devices such as rhymes, songs, and stories.

DOI: 10.4018/978-1-6684-7828-8.ch006

INTRODUCTION

Traditional Chinese medicine students find pharmacology challenging because it is complicated, yet they still need to understand facts about the mechanism of actions of drugs and how to use this knowledge in clinical settings.

Mnemonics are strategies that can enhance learning and memory of course material. Mnemonics are memory techniques that aid in chunking and organizing material to be learnt; as a result, they improve encoding and ease retrieval. There are variety of forms that include acronyms and acrostics (also known as first-letter mnemonics), the loci method, the peg word method, the keyword approach, auditory, visual, and kinesthetic mnemonics, and a group of semantic-based mnemonic devices such as rhymes, songs, and stories.

Bian et al. (2020) mentioned the importance of mnemonics in the complex medical topics such as Cardiac cycle. The authors agreed that it can be challenging for teachers to teach Cardiac cycle with a Wiggers diagram to undergraduate students, because it is difficult for them to understand since it contains a large amount of information. In their study, they concluded that, simple mnemonic could make a didactic lecture more effective.

A study conducted on 481 undergraduates who were currently enrolled in, or had taken, at least one college-level psychology course was recruited and found the ratings for mnemonics were positive and correlated with independent measures of metacognition (McCabe et al., 2013). The other study, involved 159 students of undergraduate courses as well as medical and dentistry faculties of the Golestan University of Medical Sciences in Iran demonstrated that the hand mnemonics, a type of visual mnemonics was useful and provided better insights into ion channel gating for them (Hosseini, 2018).

As described in the literature, the role of mnemonics in medical education and practice is undeniable with the fact that there are plenty of publications about this topic worldwide (Lewis Jr., et al., 2018).

In this chapter, we are going to introduce mnemonic to understand the adverse drug effects.

MNEMONIC AND UNDERSTANDING ADVERSE EFFECTS OF DRUGS

The term "cholinergic agonists" refers to a class of drugs that function in a manner similar to acetylcholine (Pakala et al., 2022). One of the most prevalent neurotransmitters in the human body, acetylcholine affects both the central and peripheral neural systems. The authors propose a mnemonic, to memorize adverse effects observed with cholinergic agonist "*MUD-DN*," which includes Miosis, Urinary urgency, Diarrhea, Diaphoresis, Nausea (Harvey et al., 2011). To memorize it easily the authors proposed the acronym as "*Magnificent Union of Digitally Downloading Nature*" or "*MUD DAY NIGHT*". The authors suggested to students to memorize "MUD DAY NIGHT," as a phrase to a widely used mnemonic. Cholinergic agonist has been clinically indicated to treat Alzheimer's disease, glaucoma, paralytic ileus, urinary retention, and myasthenia gravis (Patil & Upaganlawar, 2020). The component of "*MUD-DN*" has been given in Table 1.

Table 1. Components of "MUD-DN"

Alphabets	Adverse Effects Observed With Cholinergic Agonist
M	Miosis
U	Urinary urgency
D	Diarrhoea
D	Diaphoresis
N	Nausea

Magnificent Union of Digitally Downloading Nature

The term "cholinergic antagonist" refers to substances that bind to nicotinic or muscarinic acetylcholine receptors but prevent the normal intracellular signaling pathways from being activated. The authors proposes a mnemonic, to memorize adverse effects observed with cholinergic antagonist "*MB-CCU*", which includes mydriasis, blurred vision, confusion, constipation, urinary retention (Harvey et al., 2011). To memorize it easily the authors proposed the acronym as "*May Be Completely Considered Unnecessary*" The authors suggested to students to memorize the acronym as a phrase to a widely used mnemonic. The component of "*MB-CCU*" has been given in Table 2.

Table 2. Components of "MB-CCU"

Alphabets	Component of Acronym	Adverse Effects Observed With Cholinergic Antagonist
M	May	Miosis
B	Be	Urinary urgency
C	Completely	Diarrhea
C	Considered	Diaphoresis
U	Unnecessary	Nausea

May Be Completely Considered Unnecessary

The adrenergic drugs affect receptors that are stimulated by norepinephrine or epinephrine (Bhandari, 2018). The α-2 adrenergic receptor agonists have been used for decades to treat common medical conditions such as hypertension; attention-deficit/hyperactivity disorder; various pain and panic disorders; symptoms of opioid, benzodiazepine, and alcohol withdrawal; and cigarette craving (Giovannitti et al., 2015). The researcher proposes a mnemonic, to memorize adverse effects observed with adrenergic agonist "*ANTI-HH*", which includes Arrhythmias, Nausea, Tremors, Insomnia, Headache, Hyperactivity (Harvey et al., 2011). To memorize it easily the authors proposed the acronym as "*ANTI-HERO*" The authors suggested to students to memorize the acronym as a phrase to a widely used mnemonic. The component of *"ANTI-HH"* has been given in Table 3.

Table 3. Components of "ANTI-HH"

Alphabets	Adverse Effects Observed With Adrenergic Agonist
A	Arrhythmias
N	Nausea
T	Tremors
I	Insomnia
H	Headache
H	Hyperactivity

ANTI-Hero

Alpha-blockers are medications used in the management and treatment of essential hypertension, benign prostatic hyperplasia (BPH), and pheochromocytoma (Miller & Cumpston, 2014). The authors propose a mnemonic, to memorize some adverse effects observed with α-nonselective adrenergic blocking agents *"TVOS"*, which includes Tachycardia, Vertigo, Orthostatic Hypotension and Sexual dysfunction (Harvey et al., 2011). To memorize it easily the authors proposed the acronym as *"Treasure Valley Orchid Society"*. The authors suggested to students to memorize *"Treasure Valley Orchid Society",* as a phrase to a widely used mnemonic. The acronym has been inspired from the Treasure Valley Orchid Society, that was founded in 1971 by a dedicated group of orchid enthusiasts who came together to share their knowledge (Anonymous, 2022d). The component of *"TVOS"* has been given in Table 4.

Table 4. Components of "TVOS"

Alphabets	Component of Acronym	Some Adverse Effects Commonly Observed With Nonselective α-Adrenergic Blocking Agents
T	Treasure	Tachycardia
V	Valley	Vertigo
O	Orchid	Orthostatic hypotension
S	Society	Sexual dysfunction

Treasure Valley Orchid Society

Propranolol can be used for migraine prophylaxis, restless leg syndrome, tachyarrhythmias, acute ischemic attack prevention, and angina to reduce the sympathetic response (Shahrokhi & Gupta, 2022). The authors propose a mnemonic, to memorize some adverse effects observed in individuals treated with propranolol *"FBSA"*, which includes Fatigue, Bronchoconstriction, Sexual dysfunction and Arrhythmias (Harvey et al., 2011). To memorize it easily the authors proposed the acronym as *"Frisco Baseball and Softball Association"*. The authors suggested to students to memorize *"Frisco Baseball and Softball Association"*, as a phrase to a widely used mnemonic. The acronym has been inspired from the *Frisco Baseball Softball Association* ("FBSA") which is an ALL VOLUNTEER, non-profit organization committed to providing the youth with a positive and rewarding baseball experience (Anonymous, 2022b). The component of *"FBSA"* has been given in Table 5.

Table 5. Components of "FBSA"

Alphabets	Component of Acronym	Adverse Effects Commonly Observed In Individuals Treated With Propranolol
F	Frisco	Fatigue
B	Baseball	Bronchoconstriction
S	Softball	Sexual dysfunction
A	Association	Arrhythmias

Frisco Baseball and Softball Association

Levodopa is a dopamine precursor used in the management of Parkinson's disease, often in combination with carbidopa, as well as other conditions associated with parkinsonism (Djamshidian & Poewe, 2016). The authors propose a mnemonic, to memorize some adverse effects of levodopa *"ANHTP"*, which includes Anorexia, Nausea, Hypotension, Tachycardia and Psychiatric problems (Harvey et al., 2011). To memorize it easily the authors proposed the acronym as *"ANNA Has The Parkinson's disease"*. The authors suggested to students to memorize *"ANNA Has The Parkinson's disease"*, as a phrase to a widely used mnemonic. The phrase has been inspired from the clinical use of levodopa in the management of Parkinson's disease. The component of *"ANHTP"* has been given in Table 6.

Table 6. Components of "ANHTP"

Alphabets	Component of Acronym	Adverse Effects of Levodopa
A	ANNA	Anorexia
N		Nausea
H	Has	Hypotension
T	The	Tachycardia
P	Parkinson	Psychiatric problems

ANNA Has the Parkinson's Disease

Dopamine agonists (DA) are therapeutic agents that are commonly used in the treatment of Parkinson's disease (PD) (Borovac, 2016). The authors propose a mnemonic, to memorize some adverse effects of dopamine agonist *"SH-CNH"*, which includes Sedation, Hallucination, Confusion, Nausea, Hypotension (Harvey et al., 2011). To memorize it easily the authors proposed the acronym as *"Safety and Health Council of New Hampshire"*. The authors suggested to students to memorize *"Safety and Health Council of New Hampshire"*, as a phrase to a widely used mnemonic. The component of *"SHCNH"* has been given in Table 7.

Table 7. Components of "SH-CNH"

Alphabets	Component of Acronym	Some Adverse Effects of Dopamine Agonists
S	Safety	Sedation
H	Health	Hallucinations
C	Council	Confusion
N	New	Nausea
H	Hampshire	Hypotension

Safety and Health Council of New Hampshire

AChE inhibitors or anti-cholinesterases inhibit the cholinesterase enzyme from breaking down ACh, increasing both the level and duration of the neurotransmitter action (Colovic et al., 2013). The authors propose a mnemonic, to memorize some adverse effects of acetylcholineasterase inhibitor *"TNB-DAM"*, which includes Tremors, Nausea, Bradycardia, Diarrhea, Anorexia, Myalgia (Harvey et al., 2011). To memorize it easily the authors proposed the acronym as *"This Nosebleed Damn"*. The authors suggested to students to memorize *"This Nosebleed Damn"*, as a phrase to a widely used mnemonic. They are used in the treatment of Alzheimer's Disease and Organophosphates Induced Intoxication (Colovic et al., 2013). The component of *"TNB-DAM"* has been given in Table 8.

Table 8. Components of "TNB-DAM"

Alphabets	Component of Acronym	Adverse Effects of Acetylcholinesterase Inhibitors
T	The	Tremors
N	Nose	Nausea
B	Bleed	Bradycardia
D	Damn	Diarrhoea
A		Anorexia
M		Myalgia

This Nosebleed Damn

Barbiturates are a group of sedative-hypnotic medications used for the treatment of seizure disorder, neonatal withdrawal, insomnia, preoperative anxiety, induction of coma for increased intracranial pressure. They are also useful for inducing anesthesia (Nobay & Acquisto, 2014). The authors propose a mnemonic, to memorize some adverse effects of barbiturates *"POV-DENT"*, which includes Potential for addiction, Vertigo, Drowsiness, Enzyme induction, Nausea and Tremors (Harvey et al., 2011). To memorize it easily the authors proposed the acronym as *"Point of View on DENT"*. The authors suggested to students to memorize *"Point of View on DENT"*, as a phrase to a widely used mnemonic. The component of *"POV-DENT"* has been given in Table 9.

Table 9. Components of "POV-DENT"

Alphabets	Component of Acronym	Adverse Effects of Barbiturates
P	Point	Potential for addiction
V	View	Vertigo
D	DENT	Drowsiness
E		Enzyme induction
N		Nausea
T		Tremors

Point of View on DENT

The most often prescribed group of drugs, known as SSRIs, is used to treat depression. Due to their safety, effectiveness, and tolerability, they are frequently used as first-line pharmacotherapy for depression and many other mental illnesses (Ogata et al., 2019). The authors propose a mnemonic, to memorize some commonly observed adverse effects of selective serotonin reuptake inhibitors *"NAD-IS"*, which includes Nausea, Anxiety, Drowsiness, Insomnia, Sexual Dysfunction (Harvey et al., 2011). To memorize it easily the authors proposed the acronym as *"National Animal Disease Information Service"*. The authors suggested to students to memorize *"National Animal Disease Information Service"*, as a phrase to a widely used mnemonic. The phrase has been inspired from the NADIS (The National Animal Disease Information Service), that was formed by livestock vets in 1995 to promote animal health and welfare through improved disease prevention delivered by active veterinary health planning (Anonymous, 2022c). The component of *"NADIS"* has been given in Table 10.

Table 10. Components of "NAD-IS"

Alphabets	Component of Acronym	Some Commonly Observed Adverse Effects of Selective Serotonin Reuptake Inhibitors
N	National	Nausea
A	Animal	Anxiety
D	Disease	Drowsiness
I	Information	Insomnia
S	System	Sexual dysfunction

National Animal Disease Information Service

Tricyclic antidepressants are a class of medications used in the management and treatment of major depressive disorder (Crowell-Davis, 2019). The authors propose a mnemonic, to memorize some commonly observed adverse effects of tricyclic antidepressants *"WD-CUT-BAND"*, which includes Weight gain, Dry Mouth, Constipation, Urinary retention, Tachycardia, Blurred vision, Arrhythmias, Nausea, Drowsiness (Harvey et al., 2011). To memorize it easily the authors proposed the acronym as *"Western District Cricket Union Team BAND"*. The authors suggested to students to memorize *Western District Cricket Union Team BAND"*, as a phrase to a widely used mnemonic. The component of *"WD-CUT-BAND"* has been given in Table 11.

Table 11. Components of "WD-CUT-BAND"

Alphabets	Component of Acronym	Some Commonly Observed Adverse Effects of Tricyclic Antidepressants
W	West	Weight gain
D	District	Dry mouth
C	Cricket	Constipation
U	Union	Urinary retention
T	Team	Tachycardia
B	BAND	Blurred vision
A		Arrhythmias
N		Nausea
D		Drowsiness

Western District Cricket Union Team Band

Antipsychotic medications are mainstays in the treatment of schizophrenia and a range of other psychotic disorders such as schizoaffective disorder, delusional disorder and bipolar affective disorder (Lally & MacCabe, 2015). The authors propose a mnemonic, to memorize some commonly observed adverse effects of tricyclic antidepressants *"UWS-SEP-SAD"*, which includes Urinary retention, Weight gain, Seizure, Sedation, Extrapyramidal symptoms, Postural hypotension, Sexual Dysfunction, Arrhythemias, and Dry mouth (Harvey et al., 2011). To memorize it easily the authors proposed the acronym as *"University of Wisconsin System in September is SAD"*. The authors suggested to students to memorize *"University of Wisconsin System in September is SAD"*, as a phrase to a widely used mnemonic. The component of *"UWS-SEP-SAD"* has been given in Table 12.

Table 12. Components of "UWS-SEP-SAD"

Alphabets	Component of Acronym	Adverse Effects Observed in Individuals Treated With Antipsychotic Drugs
U	University	Urinary retention
W	Wisconsin	Weight Gain
S	System	Seizure
S	SEPTEMBER	Sedation
E		Extrapyramidal symptoms
P		Postural hypotension
S	SAD	Sexual dysfunction
A		Arrhythmias and sudden cardiac death
D		Dry Mouth

University of Wisconsin System in September Is SAD

Opioids are compounds that work at specific receptors in the brain to provide analgesia. Originally extracted from the sap of the poppy plant, opioids may be naturally occurring, semisynthetic, or synthetic, and their clinical activity is a function of their affinity for the opioid receptors in the brain. Opioids are useful for a wide variety of painful conditions, including acute pain, cancer pain, and chronic pain, as well as cough suppression and air hunger. However, opioid use is associated with a significant risk of addiction potential, which limits their use and contributes to the current "opioid phobia." (Trescot, 2013). The authors propose a mnemonic, to memorize adverse effects commonly observed in individuals treated with opioids *"PD-CHURNS"*, which includes Potential for addiction, Dysphoria, Constipation, Hypotension, Urinary retention, Respiratory depression, Nausea and Sedation (Harvey et al., 2011). To memorize it easily the authors proposed the acronym as *"Potential deep CHURNS"*. The authors suggested to students to memorize *"Potential deep CHURNS"*, as a phrase to a widely used mnemonic. The component of *"PD-CHURNS"* has been given in Table 13.

Table 13. Components of "PD-CHURNS"

Alphabets	Component of Acronym	Adverse Effects Commonly Observed in Individuals Treated With Opioids
P	Potential	Potential for addiction
D	Deep	Dysphoria
C	CHURNS	Constipation
H		Hypotension
U		Urinary retention
R		Respiratory depression
N		Nausea
S		Sedation

POTENTIAL DEEP CHURNS

Antiseizure medications are the mainstay of epilepsy therapy. Epilepsy is one of the most common and disabling neurologic conditions. A "seizure" is a paroxysmal alteration of neurologic function caused by the excessive, hypersynchronous discharge of neurons in the brain. "Epileptic seizure" is used to distinguish a seizure caused by abnormal neuronal firing from a nonepileptic event, such as a psychogenic seizure. Epilepsy" is the condition of recurrent, unprovoked seizures. Epilepsy has numerous causes, each reflecting underlying brain dysfunction (Stafstrom & Carmant, 2015k Shorvon et al., 2011). The authors propose a mnemonic, to memorize some adverse effects of antiseizure medications *"SA-THROWN"*, which includes sedation, ataxia, teratogencity, hponatremia, rash, osteoporosis, weight gain or weight loss, nausea, and vomiting (Harvey et al., 2011). To memorize it easily the authors proposed the acronym as *"Substance Abuse THROWN"*. The authors suggested to students to memorize *"Substance Abuse THROWN"*, as a phrase to a widely used mnemonic. The drugs involve in the treatment as abuse potential; therefore the authors have given relevant acronyms. The component of *"SA-THROWN"* has been given in Table 14.

Table 14. Components of "SA-THROWN"

Alphabets	Component of Acronym	Notable Adverse Effects of Antiseizure Medications
S	Substance	Sedation
A	Abuse	Ataxia
T	THROWN	Teratogenicity
H		Hyponatremia
R		Rash
O		Osteoporosis
W		Weight gain or weight loss
N		Nausea and Vomiting

SUBSTANCE ABUSE THROWN

Beta-blockers, as a class of drugs, are primarily used to treat cardiovascular diseases and other conditions. Beta-blockers are indicated and have FDA approval for the treatment of tachycardia, hypertension, myocardial infarction, congestive heart failure, cardiac arrhythmias, coronary artery disease, hyperthyroidism, essential tremor, aortic dissection, portal hypertension, glaucoma, migraine prophylaxis, and other conditions (Farzam & Jan, 2018). The authors propose a mnemonic, to memorize some adverse effects of β-blockers *"B-FISH"*, which includes Bradycardia, Fatigue, Insomnia, Sexual dysfunction and Hypotension (Harvey et al., 2011). To memorize it easily the authors proposed the acronym as *"Beautiful FISH"*. The authors suggested to students to memorize *"Beautiful FISH"*, as a phrase to a widely used mnemonic. The component of *"B-FISH"* has been given in Table 15.

Table 15. Components of "B-FISH"

Alphabets	Component of Acronym	Some Adverse Effects of β-Blockers
B	Beautiful	Bradycardia
F	FISH	Fatigue
I		Insomnia
S		Sexual dysfunction
H		Hypotension

Beautiful FISH

Calcium channel antagonists, also known as calcium channel blockers (CCBs), have been widely used for hypertension, coronary spasm, angina pectoris, supraventricular dysrhythmias, hypertrophic cardiomyopathy, and pulmonary hypertension. In addition to these, they are also prescribed for Raynaud phenomenon, subarachnoid hemorrhage, and migraine headaches (Taddei & Bruno, 2019). The authors propose a mnemonic, to memorize some common adverse effects of the calcium-channel blockers *"FH-HDFC"*, which includes Flushing, Headache, Hypotension, Dizziness, Fatigue and Constipation (Harvey et al., 2011). To memorize it easily the authors proposed the acronym as *"Family History of Heavy Drinking in Football Club"*. The authors suggested to students to memorize *"Family History of Heavy Drinking in Football Club"*, as a phrase to a widely used mnemonic. The component of *"FH-HDFC"* has been given in Table 16.

Table 16. Components of "FH-HDFC"

Alphabets	Component of Acronym	Some Common Adverse Effects of the Calcium-Channel Blockers
F	Family	Flushing
H	History	Headache
H	Heavy	Hypotension
D	Drinking	Dizziness
F	Football	Fatigue
C	Club	Constipation

Family History of Heavy Drinking in Football Club

Loop diuretics are medications used in the management and treatment of fluid overload conditions such as heart failure, nephrotic syndrome or cirrhosis, and hypertension, in addition to edema (Huxel et al., 2022). The authors propose a mnemonic, to memorize some adverse effects observed with loop diuretics *"O-HHHH"*, which includes Ototoxicity, Hyperuricemia, Hypotension, Hypemagnesemia (Harvey et al., 2011). To memorize it easily the authors proposed the acronym as *"OHHHH"*. The adverse effect could memorize as 4H's with the addition of letter "O". The component of *"O-HHHH"* has been given in Table 17.

Table 17. Components of "O-HHHH"

Alphabets	Component of Acronym	Summary of Some Adverse Effects Commonly Observed With Loop Diuretics
O	OHHHH	Ototoxicity
H		Hyperuricemia
H		Hypotension
H		Hypokalaemia
H		Hypomagnesemia

OHHHH

Insulin is commonly used in the treatment of diabetes in the home care setting. Insulin is the most effective means of lowering blood glucose, allowing the body to maintain glucose within a normal range. In people with diabetes, there is either a complete absence of this naturally occurring hormone (type 1 diabetes) or there is an issue with diminished insulin secretion and/or insulin resistance (type 2 diabetes) (Freeland & Farber, 2016). The authors propose a mnemonic, to memorize some adverse effects observed with insulin *"HATCH-LVD"*, which includes Headache, Anxiety, Tachycardia, Confusion, Hypersensitivity, Lypodystrophy, Vertigo and Diaphoresis (Harvey et al., 2011). To memorize it easily the authors proposed the acronym as *"HATCH Left ventricular dysfunction"*. The authors suggested to students to memorize *"HATCH Left ventricular dysfunction"*, as a phrase to a widely used mnemonic. In subjects with impaired glucose tolerance and patients with type 2 diabetes, insulin resistance is associated with impaired diastolic function of the left ventricle (Bajraktari et al., 2006). The component of *"HATCH-LVD"* has been given in Table 18.

Table 18. Components of "HATCH-LVD"

Alphabets	Component of Acronym	Adverse Effects Observed With Insulin
H	HATCH	Headache
A		Anxiety
T		Tachycardia
C		Confusion
H		Hypersensitivity
L	LEFT VENTRICULAR DYSFUNCTION	Lipodystrophy
V		Vertigo
D		Diaphoresis

HATCH Left Ventricular Dysfunction

The most effective management of diabetes mellitus demands an interprofessional approach involving both lifestyle modifications with diet and exercise and pharmacologic therapies as necessary to meet individualized glycemic goals. Lifestyle modifications must be combined with oral pharmacologic agents for optimal glycemic control, particularly as type 2 diabetes mellitus progresses with continued loss of pancreatic beta-cell function and insulin production (Ganesan et al., 2022). The authors propose a mnemonic, to memorize some adverse effects observed with oral hypoglycemic agents *"HG-NCW"*, which includes Hypoglycemic, Gastrointestinal disturbance, Nausea, Cardiovascular Risk and Weight gain (Harvey et al., 2011). To memorize it easily the authors proposed the acronym as *"Holland Germany New Zealand Canada Wales"*. The authors suggested to students to memorize *"Holland Germany New Zealand Canada Wales"* as a phrase to a widely used mnemonic. The component of *"HG-NCW"* has been given in Table 6.

Table 19. Components of "HG-NCW"

Alphabets	Component of Acronym	Some Adverse Effects Observed With Oral Hypoglycemic Agents
H	Holland	Hypoglycaemic
G	Germany	Gastrointestinal disturbance
N	New-Zealand	Nausea
C	Canada	Cardiovascular risk
W	Wales	Weight gain

Holland, Germany, New Zealand, Canada, Wales

Menopause is associated with a marked decrease in ovarian estrogen production. Hormone replacement therapy (HRT) is the most commonly used treatment for managing menopausal symptoms and has been shown to be the most effective intervention (Hamoda et al., 2020). The authors propose a mnemonic, to memorize some adverse effects associated with estrogen therapy *"HTN-MH-P"*, which includes Hypertension, Thromboembolism, Nausea, Myocardial Infarction, Headache and Peripheral edema (Harvey et al., 2011). To memorize it easily the authors proposed the acronym as *"Hypertension when drive in Missouri State Highway Patrol"*. The authors suggested to students to memorize *"Hypertension when drive in Missouri*

State Highway Patrol", as a phrase to a widely used mnemonic. The component of *"HTN-MH-P"* has been given in Table 20.

Table 20. Components of "HTN-MH-P"

Alphabets	Component of Acronym	Some Adverse Effects Associated With Estrogen Therapy
H	Hypertension	Hypertension
T		Thromboembolism
N		Nausea
M	Missouri state	Myocardial Infarction
H	Highway	Headache
P	Patrol	Peripheral edema

Hypertension When Driving in Missouri State Highway Patrol

Progestin preparations are made of synthetic progesterone and have often been used for hormone therapy in gynecological patients with endometriosis or endometrial cancer. Hormone therapy using progestin is considered to be one of the effective means of treatment particularly when dealing with endometrial cancer (an estrogen-dependent tumor) (Banno, 2012). The authors propose a mnemonic, to memorize some adverse effects associated with progestin therapy *"DWCH"*, which includes Depression, Weight gain, Change in Libido and Headache (Harvey et al., 2011). To memorize it easily the authors proposed the acronym as *"Detroit Wayne County Health Authority"*. The authors suggested to students to memorize *"Detroit Wayne County Health Authority"*, as a phrase to a widely used mnemonic. The phrase has been inspired from the Detroit Wayne County Health Authority, or Authority Health, which is a public body corporate that was created by the State of Michigan, Wayne County, and City of Detroit to support the public health infrastructure and create a community health network (Anonymous, 2022a). The component of *"DWCH"* has been given in Table 21.

Table 21. Components of "DWCH"

Alphabets	Component of Acronym	Some Adverse Effects Associated With Progestin Therapy
D	Detroit	Depression
W	Wayne	Weight gain
C	County	Change in Libido
H	Health authority	Headache

Detroit Wayne County Health Authority

Proton pump inhibitor therapy are irreplaceable drugs in the management of acid-related diseases (Scarpignato et al., 2016). The authors propose a mnemonic, to memorize some adverse effects of proton pump therapy *"G-NBDH"*, which includes GI Disturbance, Nausea, Bone Fraction, Diarhoea and Headache (Harvey et al., 2011). To memorize it easily the authors proposed the acronym as *"Give National Board Dental Hygiene Examination"*. The authors suggested to students to memorize *"Give National Board Dental Hygiene Examination"*, as a phrase to a widely used mnemonic. The phrase has been inspired from National Board Dental Hygiene Examination in U.S. The component of *"G-NBDH"* has been given in Table 22.

Table 22. Components of "G-NBDH"

Alphabets	Component of Acronym	Some Adverse Effects of Proton Pump Therapy
G	Give	GI disturbance
N	National	Nausea
B	Board	Bone Fractures
D	Dental	Diarrhoea
H	Hygiene examination	Headache

Give National Board Dental Hygiene Examination

The penicillin family is one of the most valuable groups of antibiotics in primary care. They are bacteriocidal, well distributed, and highly efficacious against susceptible organisms (E. L. Miller, 2002). The authors propose a mnemonic, to memorize some adverse effects of penicillin *"HHNN-DC"*, which includes Hypersensitivity, Hematologic toxicities, Nephritis, Neurotoxicity, Diarrhea and Cation Toxicity (Harvey et al., 2011). To memorize it easily the authors proposed the acronym as

"Houten Hart Noord Nederland District of Columbia". The authors suggested to students to memorize *"Houten Hart Noord Nederland District of Columbia"*, as a phrase to a widely used mnemonic. The component of *"HHNN-DC"* has been given in Table 23.

Table 23. Components of "HHNN-DC"

Alphabets	Component of Acronym	Summary of the Adverse Effects of Penicillin
H	Houten	Hypersensitivity
H	Hart	Hematologic toxicities
N	Noord	Nephritis
N	Nederland	Neurotoxicity
D	District	Diarrhea
C	of Columbia	Cation toxicity

Houten Hart Noord Nederland District of Columbia

Tetracyclines were discovered in the 1940s and exhibited activity against a wide range of microorganisms including gram-positive and gram-negative bacteria, chlamydiae, mycoplasmas, rickettsiae, and protozoan parasites. They are inexpensive antibiotics, which have been used extensively in the prophlylaxis and therapy of human and animal infections and also at subtherapeutic levels in animal feed as growth promoters (Chopra & Roberts, 2001). The authors propose a mnemonic, to memorize some adverse effects of tetracycline *"GDLP-VA"*, which includes GI-Disturbance, Deposition of drug in bones and teeth, Liver failure, Phototoxicity, Vertigo and Avoid in pregnancy (Harvey et al., 2011). To memorize it easily the authors proposed the acronym as *"Graduated Drivers Licensing Program in Valencia"*. The authors suggested to students to memorize *"Graduated Drivers Licensing Program in Valencia"*, as a phrase to a widely used mnemonic. The component of *"GDLP-VA"* has been given in Table 24.

Table 24. Components of "GDLP-VA"

Alphabets	Component of Acronym	Some Adverse Effects of Tetracyclines
G	Graduated	GI disturbance
D	Drivers	Deposition of drug in bones and teeth
L	Licensing	Liver failure
P	Program	Phototoxicity
V	Valencia	Vertigo
A		Avoid in Pregnancy

Graduated Driver Licensing Program in Valencia

Aminoglycosides are rapidly bactericidal, concentration dependent antibiotics with a broad spectrum of activity against Gram-negative and Gram-positive organisms, including those that are multidrug resistant (MDR). Overall, the class has potent activity against Enterobacteriaceae family members and is less active against Pseudomonas aeruginosa and Acinetobacter spp (Sader et al., 2015a, 2015b).The authors propose a mnemonic, to memorize some adverse effects of aminoglycosides *"ONPS"*, which includes Ototoxicity, Nephrotoxicty, Paralysis and Skin rashes (Harvey et al., 2011). To memorize it easily the authors proposed the acronym as *"Oklahoma Native Plant Society"*. The authors suggested to students to memorize *"Oklahoma Native Plant Society"*, as a phrase to a widely used mnemonic. The phrase has been inspired from Oklahoma Native Plant Society. The student can memorize the adverse effect by memorizing *"PONS"* which is pons is a part of brainstem, a structure that links your brain to your spinal cord. It handles unconscious processes and jobs, such as your sleep-wake cycle and breathing. The component of *"ONPS"* has been given in Table 25.

Table 25. Components of "ONPS"

Alphabets	Component of Acronym	Some Adverse Effects of Aminoglycosides
O	Oklahoma	Ototoxicity
N	Native	Nephrotoxicity
P	Plant	Paralysis
S	Society	Skin rashes

Oklahoma Native Plant Society

Macrolides are a class of drugs used to manage and treat various bacterial infections. Azithromycin, clarithromycin, and erythromycin are commonly used to treat infections like pneumonia, sinusitis, pharyngitis, and tonsillitis. They are also used in uncomplicated skin infections and otitis media in pediatric patients. Clarithromycin is used to treat Helicobacter pylori infections in standard triple therapy protocol regardless of clarithromycin resistance status. Macrolides are also commonly used to treat sexually transmitted infections such as gonococcal and chlamydial infections (Patel & Hashmi, 2022). The authors propose a mnemonic, to memorize some adverse effects of macrolide *"JOG"*, which includes Jaundice, Ototoxicity, GI Disturbance (Harvey et al., 2011). The component of *"JOG"* has been given in Table 26.

Table 26. Components of "JOG"

Alphabets	Component of Acronym	Some Adverse Effects of Macrolide Antibiotics
J	JOG	Jaundice
O		Ototoxicity
G		GI disturbance

JOG

The fluoroquinolones are a family of broad spectrum, systemic antibacterial agents that have been used widely as therapy of respiratory and urinary tract infections. Fluoroquinolones are active against a wide range of aerobic gram-positive and gram-negative organisms. Gram-positive coverage includes penicillinase- and non-penicillinase producing Staphylococci, Streptococcus pneumoniae and viridans, Enterococcus faecalis, Listeria monocytogenes, and Nocardia species. Gram negative coverage includes Neisseria meningitides and gonorrhoeae, Haemophilus influenzae, and most clinically important Enterobacteriaceae species, Pseudomonas aeruginosa and Vibrio species (Anonymous, 2012). The authors propose a mnemonic, to memorize some adverse effects of fluoroquinolones *"DNN-HD"*, which includes Dizziness, Diarrhea, Nausea, Nephrotoxicity and Headache (Harvey et al., 2011). To memorize it easily the authors proposed the acronym as *"Deep Neural Network Hashing"*. The authors suggested to students to memorize *"Deep Neural Network Hashing"*, as a phrase to a widely used mnemonic. The component of *"DNN-HD"* has been given in Table 27.

Table 27. Components of "DNN-HD"

Alphabets	Component of Acronym	Some Adverse Reactions to Fluoroquinolones
D	Deep	Dizziness
D		Diarrhoea
N	Neural	Nausea
N	Network	Nephrotoxicity
H	Hashing	Headache

Deep Neural Network Hashing

Sulfonamides have been in clinical use for many years, and the development of bioactive substances containing the sulfonamide subunit has grown steadily in view of their important biological properties such as antibacterial, antifungal, antiparasitic, antioxidant, and antitumour properties (Azevedo-Barbosa et al., 2020). The authors propose a mnemonic, to memorize some adverse effects of sulphonamides *"CHHC"*, which includes Crystalluria, Hypersensitivity, Hemolytic anemia, and CNS effects (Harvey et al., 2011). To memorize it easily the authors proposed the acronym as *Certified Holistic Health Coach"*. The authors suggested to students to memorize *"Certified Holistic Health Coach"*, as a phrase to a widely used mnemonic. The component of *"CHHC"* has been given in Table 28.

Table 28. Components of "CHHC"

Alphabets	Component of Acronym	Some Adverse Reactions to Sulphonamides
C	Certified	Crystalluria
H	Holistic	Hypersensitivity
H	Health	Hemolytic anemia
C	Coach	CNS effects

Certified Holistic Health Coach

Metronidazole is one of the mainstay drugs for the treatment of anaerobic bacterial infections, protozoal infections, and microaerophilic bacterial infections. It is cytotoxic to facultative anaerobic microorganisms. It is used to treat intestinal amebiases, liver amebiasis, bacterial septicemia, bone and joint infections, meningitis, brain abscess, endocarditis, endometritis, bacterial vaginosis, intra-abdominal infections, lower respiratory tract infections, skin structure infections, and surgical prophylaxis colorectal surgeries (Weir & Le, 2022). The authors propose a mnemonic, to memorize some adverse effects of metronidazole *"NGM"*, which includes Nausea, GI Disturbance and Metallic taste (Harvey et al., 2011). To memorize it easily the authors proposed the acronym as *"National Geographic Magazine"*. The authors suggested to students to memorize *"National Geographic Magazine"*, as a phrase to a widely used mnemonic. The component of *"MGM"* has been given in Table 29.

Table 29. Components of "NGM"

Alphabets	Component of Acronym	Adverse Effects of Metronidazole
N	National	Nausea
G	Geographic	GI disturbance
M	Magazine	Metallic taste

National Geographic Magazine

Chloroquine is well known anti-malarial drug. The authors propose a mnemonic, to memorize some adverse effects of chloroquine *"GSHB"*, which includes GI Disturbance, Skin rashes, Headache, Blurred vision (Harvey et al., 2011). To memorize it easily the authors proposed the acronym as *"Genome Systems Human BAC (Bacterial Artificial Chromosome)"*. The authors suggested to students to memorize *"Genome Systems Human BAC (Bacterial Artificial Chromosome)"*, as a phrase to a widely used mnemonic. The component of *"GSHB"* has been given in Table 30.

Table 30. Components of "GSHB"

Alphabets	Component of Acronym	Some Adverse Effects Commonly Associated With Chloroquine
G	Genome	GI disturbance
S	Systems	Skin rash
H	Human	Headache
B	Bacterial artificial chromosome	Blurred vision

Genome Systems Human BAC (Bacterial Artificial Chromosome)

Efavirenz is an antiretroviral medication used to treat and prevent HIV/AIDS (Dai et al., 2019). The authors propose a mnemonic, to memorize some adverse effects of efavirenz *"NDV"*, which includes Not during Pregnancy, Dizziness and Vivid dreams (Harvey et al., 2011). To memorize it easily the authors proposed the acronym as *"Newcastle Disease Virus"*. The authors suggested to students to memorize *"Newcastle Disease Virus"*, as a phrase to a widely used mnemonic. The phrase has been inspired from the Newcastle disease (ND), which is a highly contagious and often severe disease found worldwide that affects birds including domestic poultry. It is caused by virulent strains of avian paramyxovirus type 1. The component of *"NDV"* has been given in Table 31.

Table 31. Components of "NDV"

Alphabets	Component of Acronym	Adverse Reactions of Efavirenz
N	Newcastle	Not during Pregnancy
D	Disease	Dizziness
V	Virus	Vivid dreams

Newcastle Disease Virus

The authors propose a mnemonic, to memorize some adverse effects of iloprost *"DHFF"*, which includes Dizziness, Headache, Flushing and Fainting (Harvey et al., 2011). To memorize it easily the authors proposed the acronym as *"Directorate of Horticulture and Field Forestry"*. The authors suggested to students to memorize *"Directorate of Horticulture and Field Forestry"*, as a phrase to a widely used mnemonic. The component of *"DHFF"* has been given in Table 32.

Table 32. Components of "DHFF"

Alphabets	Component of Acronym	Some Adverse Reactions to Iloprost
D	Directorate	Dizziness
H	Horticulture	Headache
F	Field	Flushing
F	Forestry	Fainting

Directorate of Horticulture and Field Forestry

Aspirin is a non-steroidal anti-inflammatory drug that is an irreversible inhibitor of both cyclooxygenase (COX)-1 and COX-2, It stimulates endogenous production of anti-inflammatory regulatory 'braking signals', including lipoxins, which dampen the inflammatory response and reduce levels of inflammatory biomarkers, including C-reactive protein, tumor necrosis factor-α and interleukin (IL)--6, but not negative immunoregulatory cytokines, such as IL-4 and IL-10. Aspirin can reduce oxidative stress and protect against oxidative damage. Early evidence suggests there are beneficial effects of aspirin in preclinical and clinical studies in mood disorders and schizophrenia, and epidemiological data suggests that high-dose aspirin is associated with a reduced risk of Alzheimer's disease (AD) (Berk et al., 2013). The authors propose a mnemonic, to memorize some adverse effects of aspirin *"R-HRGP"*, which includes Reye syndrome, Hypersensitivity, Respiratory depression, GI disturbance and Prolonged bleeding time (Harvey et al., 2011). To memorize it easily the authors proposed the acronym as *"Rise, Hire and Retain Good People"*. The authors suggested to students to memorize *"Rise, Hire and Retain Good People"*, as a phrase to a widely used mnemonic. The component of *"R-HRGP"* has been given in Table 33.

Table 33. Components of "R-HRGP"

Alphabets	Component of Acronym	Some Adverse Reactions to Aspirin
R	Rise	Reye syndrome
H	Hire	Hypersensitivity
R	Retain	Respiratory depression
G	Good	GI disturbance
P	People	Prolonged bleeding time

Rise, Hire, and Retain Good People

The authors propose a mnemonic, to memorize some adverse effects of colchicine *"GONAAD"*, which includes GI Disturbance, Nausea, Alopecia, Aplastic anemia and diarrhea (Harvey et al., 2011). The component of *"GONAAD"* has been given in Table 34.

Table 34. Components of "GONAAD"

Alphabets	Component of Acronym	Some Adverse Effects of Colchicine
G	GONAAD	GI Disturbance
N		Nausea
A		Alopecia
A		Aplastic anemia
D		Diarrhea

GONAAD

H1-antihistamines are inverse agonists that combine with and stabilize inactive conformation of H1-receptors. Thus, they interfere with actions of histamine at H1-receptors. They are widely used for treatment of allergic rhinitis, allergic conjunctivitis, urticaria, coughs, colds and insomnia (Kalpaklioglu & Baccioglu, 2012).The authors propose a mnemonic, to memorize some adverse effects of levodopa *"HD-VD-UTI"*, which includes Hypotension, Drowsiness, Vertigo, Dry Mouth, Urinary Retention, Tachycardia and increased appetite (Harvey et al., 2011). To memorize it easily the authors proposed the acronym as *"High-Definition Video Urinary tract infection"*. The authors suggested to students to memorize *"High-Definition Video Urinary tract infection"*, as a phrase to a widely used mnemonic. The component of *"HD-VD-UTI"* has been given in Table 35.

Table 35. Components of "HD-VD-UTI"

Alphabets	Component of Acronym	Some Adverse Effects Observed With First-Generation H1 Antihistamines
H	High Definition	Hypotension
D		Drowsiness
V	Video	Vertigo
D		Dry mouth
U	Urinary tract infection	Urinary retention
T		Tachycardia
I		Increased appetite

High-Definition Video Urinary Tract Infection

Exposure to high levels of lead may cause anemia, weakness, and kidney and brain damage The authors propose a mnemonic, to memorize some adverse effects of levodopa *"FIGH"*, which includes Fatigue, Insomnia, GI Disturbance and Headache (Harvey et al., 2011). To memorize it easily the authors proposed the acronym as *"Families in Good Health"*. The authors suggested to students to memorize *"Families in Good Health"*, as a phrase to a widely used mnemonic. The component of *"FIGH"* has been given in Table 36.

Table 36. Components of "FIGH"

Alphabets	Component of Acronym	Adverse Effects of Lead Poisoning
F	Families	Fatigue
I	In	Insomnia
G	Good	GI Disturbance
H	Health	Headache

CONCLUSION

In the education of future physicians continuing, developing, and maintaining of pharmacological knowledge are crucial. The educators could help them achieving this by using mnemonics in their teaching along with didactic lecture to provide students a long-term memory of pharmacological study.

REFERENCES

Anonymous. (2012). Fluoroquinolones. In *LiverTox: Clinical and Research Information on Drug-Induced Liver Injury*. National Institute of Diabetes and Digestive and Kidney Diseases. https://www.ncbi.nlm.nih.gov/books/NBK547840/

Anonymous. (2022a). *Detroit Wayne County Health Authority*. Fostering Success Michigan. http://fosteringsuccessmichigan.com/network/detroit-wayne-county-health-authority

Anonymous. (2022b). *Frisco Baseball & Softball Association*. FBSA. https://fbsa.org/content/9226/FAQ

Anonymous. (2022c). *NADIS - National Animal Disease Information Service*. NADIS. https://www.nadis.org.uk/about/

Anonymous. (2022d). *Treasure Valley Orchid Society*. Treasure Valley. http://www.treasurevalleyorchidsociety.org/

Azevedo-Barbosa, H., Dias, D. F., Franco, L. L., Hawkes, J. A., & Carvalho, D. T. (2020). From Antibacterial to Antitumour Agents: A Brief Review on The Chemical and Medicinal Aspects of Sulfonamides. *Mini-Reviews in Medicinal Chemistry, 20*(19), 2052–2066. doi:10.2174/1389557520666200905125738 PMID:32888265

Bajraktari, G., Koltai, M. S., Ademaj, F., Rexhepaj, N., Qirko, S., Ndrepepa, G., & Elezi, S. (2006). Relationship between insulin resistance and left ventricular diastolic dysfunction in patients with impaired glucose tolerance and type 2 diabetes. *International Journal of Cardiology, 110*(2), 206–211. doi:10.1016/j.ijcard.2005.08.033 PMID:16297997

Banno, K. (2012). Progestin therapy for endometrial cancer: The potential of fourth-generation progestin [Review]. *International Journal of Oncology, 40*(6), 1755–1762. doi:10.3892/ijo.2012.1384 PMID:22366992

Berk, M., Dean, O., Drexhage, H., McNeil, J. J., Moylan, S., O'Neil, A., Davey, C. G., Sanna, L., & Maes, M. (2013). Aspirin: A review of its neurobiological properties and therapeutic potential for mental illness. *BMC Medicine, 11*(1), 1–17. doi:10.1186/1741-7015-11-74 PMID:23506529

Bhandari, P. (2018). Adrenergic Drugs. In Pharmacology for Medical Undergraduates (pp. 67–67). Jaypee Brothers Medical Publishers (P) Ltd. doi:10.5005/jp/books/14244_9

Bian, H., Bian, Y., Li, J., Xu, S., Shao, X., Li, J., & Jiang, B. (2020, March 1). A simple hand mnemonic for teaching the cardiac cycle. *Advances in Physiology Education, 44*(1), 21–25. doi:10.1152/advan.00059.2019 PMID:31821034

Borovac, J. A. (2016). Side effects of a dopamine agonist therapy for Parkinson's disease: a mini-review of clinical pharmacology. *The Yale Journal of Biology and Medicine, 89*(1), 37–47.

Chopra, I., & Roberts, M. (2001). Tetracycline Antibiotics: Mode of Action, Applications, Molecular Biology, and Epidemiology of Bacterial Resistance. *Microbiology and Molecular Biology Reviews, 65*(2), 232–260. doi:10.1128/MMBR.65.2.232-260.2001 PMID:11381101

Colovic, M. B., Krstic, D. Z., Lazarevic-Pasti, T. D., Bondzic, A. M., & Vasic, V. M. (2013). Acetylcholinesterase Inhibitors: Pharmacology and Toxicology. *Current Neuropharmacology*, *11*(3), 315–335. doi:10.2174/1570159X11311030006 PMID:24179466

Crowell-Davis, S. L. (2019). Tricyclic Antidepressants. In *Veterinary Psychopharmacology* (pp. 231–256). Wiley. doi:10.1002/9781119226253.ch16

Dai, L., Liu, A., Zhang, H., Wu, H., Zhang, T., Su, B., Shao, Y., Li, J., Ye, J., Scott, S. R., Mahajan, S. D., Schwartz, S. A., Yu, H., & Sun, L. (2019). Impact of Lopinavir/Ritonavir and Efavirenz-Based Antiretroviral Therapy on the Lipid Profile of Chinese HIV/AIDS Treatment-Naïve Patients in Beijing: A Retrospective Study. *Current HIV Research*, *17*(5), 324–334. doi:10.2174/1570162X17666191025115508 PMID:31654514

Djamshidian, A., & Poewe, W. (2016). Apomorphine and levodopa in Parkinson's disease: Two revolutionary drugs from the 1950's. *Parkinsonism & Related Disorders*, *33*, S9–S12. doi:10.1016/j.parkreldis.2016.12.004 PMID:28012951

Farzam, K., & Jan, A. (2018). Drugs in Sport. In D. R. Mottram & N. Chester (Eds.), Drugs in Sport (7th ed.). Routledge. doi:10.4324/9781315222790

Freeland, B., & Farber, M. S. (2016). A Review of Insulin for the Treatment of Diabetes Mellitus. *Home Healthcare Now*, *34*(8), 416–423. doi:10.1097/NHH.0000000000000446 PMID:27580280

Ganesan, K., Rana, M. B. M., & Sultan, S. (2022). Oral Hypoglycemic Medications. In *StatPearls*. StatPearls Publishing. https://www.ncbi.nlm.nih.gov/books/NBK482386/

Giovannitti, J. A. Jr, Thoms, S. M., & Crawford, J. J. (2015). Alpha-2 Adrenergic Receptor Agonists: A Review of Current Clinical Applications. *Anesthesia Progress*, *62*(1), 31–38. doi:10.2344/0003-3006-62.1.31 PMID:25849473

Hamoda, H., Panay, N., Pedder, H., Arya, R., & Savvas, M. (2020). The British Menopause Society & Women's Health Concern 2020 recommendations on hormone replacement therapy in menopausal women. *Post Reproductive Health*, *26*(4), 181–209. doi:10.1177/2053369120957514 PMID:33045914

Harvey, R. A., Clark, M. A., Finkel, R., Rey, J. A., & Whalen, K. (2011). *Pharmacology (Lippincott's Illustrated Reviews Series)*. Lippincott Williams & Wilkins. https://books.google.com/books/about/Pharmacology.html?id=Y558dgp_PjoC

Hosseini, S. M. (2018, June 1). A useful hand mnemonic to demonstrate ion channel gating. *Advances in Physiology Education*, *42*(2), 321–323. doi:10.1152/advan.00080.2017 PMID:29676617

Huxel, C., Raja, A., & Ollivierre-Lawrence, M. D. (2022). Loop Diuretics. In *StatPearls*. StatPearls Publishing. https://www.ncbi.nlm.nih.gov/books/NBK546656/

Kalpaklioglu, F., & Baccioglu, A. (2012). Efficacy and Safety of H1-Antihistamines: An Update. *Anti-Inflammatory & Anti-Allergy Agents in Medicinal Chemistry*, *11*(3), 230–237. doi:10.2174/1871523011202030230 PMID:23173575

Lally, J., & MacCabe, J. H. (2015). Antipsychotic medication in schizophrenia: A review. *British Medical Bulletin*, *114*(1), 169–179. doi:10.1093/bmb/ldv017 PMID:25957394

Lewis, J. B. Jr, Mulligan, R., & Kraus, N. (2018). The importance of medical mnemonics in medicine. *Pharos.*, *2018*, 30–35.

McCabe, J. A., Osha, K. L., Roche, J. A., & Susser, J. A. (2013). Psychology Students' Knowledge and Use of Mnemonics. *Teaching of Psychology*, *40*(3), 183–192. doi:10.1177/0098628313487460

Miller, E. L. (2002). The Penicillins: A Review And Update. *Journal of Midwifery & Women's Health*, *47*(6), 426–434. doi:10.1016/S1526-9523(02)00330-6 PMID:12484664

Miller, S. M., & Cumpston, K. L. (2014). Alpha Blockers. In *Encyclopedia of Toxicology* (pp. 154–155). Elsevier. doi:10.1016/B978-0-12-386454-3.00714-4

Nobay, F., & Acquisto, N. M. (2014). Barbiturates. In *Encyclopedia of Toxicology* (pp. 363–367). Elsevier. doi:10.1016/B978-0-12-386454-3.00696-5

Ogata, N., Dantas, L. M., & Crowell-Davis, S. L. (2019). Selective Serotonin Reuptake Inhibitors. In *Veterinary Psychopharmacology* (pp. 103–128). Wiley. doi:10.1002/9781119226253.ch8

Pakala, R. S., Brown, K. N., & Preuss, C. V. (2022). Cholinergic Medications. In *StatPearls*. StatPearls Publishing. https://www.ncbi.nlm.nih.gov/books/NBK538163/

Patel, P. H., & Hashmi, M. F. (2022). Macrolides. In *StatPearls*. StatPearls Publishing. https://www.ncbi.nlm.nih.gov/books/NBK551495/

Patil, R., & Upaganlawar, A. (2020). Cholinergic Agonists. In *Advances in Neuropharmacology* (pp. 3–30). Apple Academic Press. doi:10.1201/9780429242717-2

Sader, H. S., Rhomberg, P. R., Farrell, D. J., & Jones, R. N. (2015). Arbekacin activity against contemporary clinical bacteria isolated from patients hospitalized with pneumonia. *Antimicrobial Agents and Chemotherapy*, *59*(6), 3263–3270. doi:10.1128/AAC.04839-14 PMID:25801559

Scarpignato, C., Gatta, L., Zullo, A., & Blandizzi, C. (2016). Effective and safe proton pump inhibitor therapy in acid-related diseases - A position paper addressing benefits and potential harms of acid suppression. *BMC Medicine*, *14*(1), 1–35. doi:10.118612916-016-0718-z PMID:27825371

ShahrokhiM.GuptaV. (2022). Propranolol. *StatPearls*. https://www.ncbi.nlm.nih.gov/books/NBK557801/

Shorvon, S. D., Andermann, F., & Guerrini, R. (2011). *The causes of epilepsy*. Cambridge University Press. doi:10.1017/CBO9780511921001

Stafstrom, C. E., & Carmant, L. (2015). Seizures and Epilepsy: An Overview for Neuroscientists. *Cold Spring Harbor Perspectives in Medicine*, *5*(6), a022426–a022426. doi:10.1101/cshperspect.a022426 PMID:26033084

Taddei, S., & Bruno, R. M. (2019). Calcium Channel Blockers. In *Encyclopedia of Endocrine Diseases* (pp. 689–695). Elsevier. doi:10.1016/B978-0-12-801238-3.65408-9

Trescot, A. (2013). Clinical Use of Opioids. In Comprehensive Treatment of Chronic Pain by Medical, Interventional, and Integrative Approaches (pp. 99–110). Springer New York. doi:10.1007/978-1-4614-1560-2_10

Weir, C. B., & Le, J. K. (2022). Metronidazole. In *StatPearls*. StatPearls Publishing. doi:10.1201/9781315152110

Chapter 7
Study on the Application of Music Memory Method in Pharmacology

Yusu Wang
Xiamen University, China

EXECUTIVE SUMMARY

Memory is the faculty by which the mind stores and remembers information. Music is some combination of vocal or instrumental sounds. Research offers new insights into how music links to memories, and how those connections make life better. Medicine is undoubtedly one of the most challenging courses for memory. In all academic settings, there is no other need for powerful mnemonic tools like medicine. In the study of pharmacology, students generally report that the course of pharmacology is difficult, some students say that the names of drugs are too complicated to remember; however, few students realize that music mnemonics is a good way to learn.

INTRODUCTION

Memory is the faculty of the mind by which data or information is encoded, stored, and retrieved when needed. It is the retention of information over time for the purpose of influencing future action. Recent research on music and brain function has suggested that the temporal pattern structure in music and rhythm can enhance cognitive functions. Song, with its memory enhancement potential and ability to engage, has been employed as a learning tool in some academic settings. Entertainment-education song has proven to be effective as a memory enhancer and learning tool across a number of disciplines.

DOI: 10.4018/978-1-6684-7828-8.ch007

Music stimulates an increase in the release of beneficial chemicals such as ethanol choline, which is thought to be a neurotransmitter that carries messages between brain cells. Therefore, the increase of ethanol choline is to enhance memory, and can promote the kinetic energy of human physiological action. In addition, music can promote metabolic activity and improve mental health. When you are upset, music will remove your worries, when you are happy, music can make you more relaxed and delighted. Listening to relaxing music regularly will keep you in an optimistic mood, you will have full of vitality, interest and confidence in life and study, which will unconsciously improve your memory.

BACKGROUND

How Music Works in Memory

Memory is the faculty by which the mind stores and remembers information. Many people compare memory to a bridge from perception to thinking. Without memory, there would be no imagination, thinking, judgment, and no way to solve problems well. Therefore, if someone wants to achieve excellent results in study, and accumulate scientific, cultural knowledge, experience, he must have a good memory, and music can help people remember. The life experiences of many celebrities have also proved that music has a very obvious effect on improving memory. The effect of music memory is often dozens of times higher than the normal memory.

Music is the vocal or instrumental sounds (or both) combined in such a way as to produce beauty of form, harmony, and expression of emotion, which is a powerful tool for getting information about yourself. Research has provided new insight into how our favorite music is linked to memory and personality, and how these connections can make life better.

When a song hasn't been sung for years, the score and lyrics are long forgotten, but just hearing the tune of that song creates a familiar, intimate feeling, and the words come to mind. The songs had a unique meaning, like the music people dance to at weddings, and improved memory performance in tests.

In Bulgaria, Russia, the U.S., France, Canada and other countries, there is a super music memory system that uses music to help memory. Dr. Lazanov of Bulgaria, based on medical and psychological research, has found that the adagio movement of Bach, Handel and others can relieve the tension in the brain and bring people into a meditative state.

He asked the students to listen to slow music and relax their muscles as they read material to the music. At the end of the study period, play upbeat music for another 2 minutes to allow the brain to recover from the memory activity. Many students who have tried this method find it very effective. Later, the Bulgarian Ministry of Education gathered more than 30 experts to establish the Razanov Institute, continue to study and constantly improve this method of learning. Students using this method were able to complete the courses in four months what would normally take a student two years before. In 1977, Mr. Razanov came to the United States and taught the method. Experiments in California, Iowa, Washington, D.C., and other places have shown that this kind of learning increases efficiency by seven times, hence the name "super mnemonics."

Research in music and education has linked songs to a variety of human traits, including memory (Hickok, Buchsbaum, Humphries, &Muftuler, 2003) speech and language acquisition (Hickok et al., 2003), Emotion (Cirigliano, 2013), intelligence (Schellenberg, 2011), and identity (Hargeaves, Miell et al., 2018). The changes were most pronounced in the prefrontal cortex, known as the brain's control center, where decision-making, social behavior regulation, personality expression and the planning of complex mental behaviors all take place.

When the people heard music that was personal to them, it powered up a musical neural network connecting different regions of the brain, based on MRIs taken of the people before and after listening to the music. This differed from when they heard new, unfamiliar music, which only triggered a specific part of the brain tuned into listening.

Overall, music looks to have found a place in every facet of life, and given its unique qualities, is certainly ripe for use in education.In fact, its roots can be traced back to the philosophers of Ancient Greece, who taught moral lessons through the dramatic arts and theatre (Piotrow, 1994).

Music in Medicine

Medicine is undoubtedly one of the most, if not the most, memory challenging courses any student can face today.

In all academic Settings, no one needs music as a learning tool as powerful as medicine. Anatomy, biochemistry, surgery, clinic, diagnosis, medicine, therapy, etc., are the basic knowledge of medical professionals. As a result, many medical students have created their own mnemonic methods to help them recall information.

In 1884, Dr. Hugo Erichsen (1860-1944) published Medical Rhymes, a collection of rhymes and illustrations from a variety of sources. "The purpose of my book," Erickson writes in the introduction, "is to entertain busy doctors in their spare time. Some serious poetry will no doubt provide thought-provoking material. Erickson himself was a busy doctor, practicing in Detroit.

This is attributed to a London medical student and is quite telling of the time, where K is for kreosote and O is for opium. This one even has a little repeating chorus.(figure 1)

Figure 1. The student's alphabet

THE STUDENT'S ALPHABET.

Oh, A was an artery, filled with injection;
And B was a brick, never caught at dissection.
C were some chemicals, lithium and borax;
D played the deuce with the bones of the thorax.

CHORUS.—

Taken in short-hand with minute accuracy.

Fol de rol lol,
Fol de rol lay,
Fol de rol, tol de rol, tol de rol, lay.

E was an embryo in a glass case;
And F a foramen that pierced the skull's base.
G was a grinder, who sharpen'd the tools;
And H means the half-and-half drunk at the schools.
Fol de rol, etc.

I was some iodine, made of sea-weed;
J was a jolly cock, not used to read.
K was some kreosote, much over-rated;
And L was the lies which about it were stated.
Fol de rol lol, etc.

M was a muscle, cold, flabby and red;
And N was a nerve, like a bit of white thread.
O was some opium, a fool chose to take;
And P were the pins used to keep him awake.
Fol de rol lol, etc.

Q was the quacks, who cure stammer and squint.
R was raw from a burn, and wrapped close in lint.
S was a scalpel, to eat bread and cheese;
And T was a tourniquet, vessels to squeeze.
Fol de rol lol, etc.

U was the unciform bone of the wrist.
V was the vein which a blunt lancet missed.
W was wax from a syringe that flowed;
X, the 'xaminers, who may be blowed!
Fol de rol lol, etc.

Y stands for you all, with best wishes sincere;
And Z for the zanies who never touch beer.
So we've got to the end, not forgetting a letter;
And those who don't like it may grind up a better.

—*London Medical Student.*

In modern society, the Internet has become a good communication platform, providing a convenient learning channel for many people. many creative pioneers have begun to explore this unexplored method of memorization and spread their own medical music memorization methods online. Student and teacher made music memorization techniques are all over the Internet, and a search for the right terms will turn up plenty of videos about them.

Let's take an example of how to use music memory to remember the cranial nerves, which is difficult but necessary for many students to remember.

The "CRANIAL NERVES SONG", published by the *Neural Academy* on the internet, aimed to teach people how to memorize not only the name of cranial nerves, but also their order, location, function and so on:

Cranial nerves emerge directly from the brain,
Unlike spinal nerves in the spinal cord's domain,
The first two cranial nerves, arise from the cerebrum
While the other ten nerves arise from the brainstem.
Your special senses are olfaction, audition vision balance gustation,
Detected by specialized organs, which collect this information.
Your general senses are temperature, vibration pressure touch and pain
Detected over a widespread area, and sent to your brain.
Cranial nerve one, the olfactory, helps you detect smells,
Transmitting signals that come from olfactory epithelium cells!
The second, the optic nerve, transmits retinal input,
This nerve allows you to see, so here it is, come look!
Pupils are constricted by the, third nerve, the oculomotor,
Also running four eye muscles, it's the eyeball's main motor.
It talks to the Edinger Westphal, and oculomotor nuclei,
To help lens accommodation, and lift the upper lid of your eye.
The fourth, the trochlear nerve, on the trochlear nucleus relies,
In order to control the superior oblique muscles of your eyes!
The fifth, the trigeminal, the largest of the cranial nerves,
Controlling mastication muscles, for chewing food it serves.
And senses temperature touch and pain, of your scalp, face, meninges,
Larynx, pharynx, sinuses, and oral and nasal cavities.
The sixth, the abducens nerve, on the abducens nucleus relies,
To innervate the lateral rectus muscles of your eyes!
The seventh, the facial nerve, feels touch behind your ear,
And controls facial expressions, like happiness or fear,

To transmitting taste from the front, 2/3 of the tongue it's devoted,
And has secretomotor function for all head glands except the parotid.
The eighth, the vestibulocochlear, this nerve has two talents,
Linking the semicircular canals, to the vestibular nucleus for balance!
And sending sound signals from cochlea to cochlear nucleus,
So it talks with two nuclei, as you'll remember if you're studious!
The ninth, the glossopharyngeal nerve, takes over the parotid gland,
Transmitting taste from the back third, of the tongue so food isn't bland,
It gives sensation to your tongue, tonsils, pharynx and eardrum too!
Innervates the stylopharyngeus muscle, measures blood pressure, pH, O2!
The tenth, the vagus nerve, has oh so many functions,
From thoracic and abdominal organs, it gets visceral sensations
It also gives sensation to your external ear.
And to your meninges, lower pharynx and larynx, here!
It innervates palate muscles, and the larynx and the pharynx,
Causes gland secretion in the, thorax, abdomen, larynx, pharynx.
The eleventh, the accessory nerve, for motor use is employed,
Innervating the upper trapezius and sternocleidomastoid!
The twelfth, the hypoglossal nerve, has motor function solely,
And innervates extrinsic and intrinsic tongue muscles totally,
Except for the palatoglossus, which elevate the tongue's back part,
And is innervated by the vagus nerve, that sets it apart!

At the bottom of the video, many people have commented on how useful the song was to them, like the account *Mehrab's Adventures* said, "Very well made. you just summarised material that takes anatomy professors months to teach! Great job!"

Of course, this isn't the only memory song about the cranial nerves. Many other people have their own unique melodies.

For example, Prof Hope (University of Nottingham Medical School) demonstrates how to remember the 12 cranial nerves, to the tune of "12 Days of Christmas", and his students recorded his songs and posted it online. "I love it! Repetition to help me learn!" *subtleXplosion* commented, "Fun movements/dances to help me remember the function! In numerical order to help me remember the order...and to top it all of, he has a present singing voice! Brilliant!"

What's more, there is an account named "learnthroughsong", it's pretty obvious from the name that this account is about using music to learn and memory, also posted a Cranial Nerves Song:

Olfactory #1, for your sense of smell
Optic nerve is #2, lets you see real well
Oculomotor, 3, lens and lids of eyes
Trochlear is #4, eyes counterclockwise
Sense skin, teeth and tongue, Trigeminal is 5
Also helps you masticate
Abducens, 6 moves eyes
Facial 7th nerve for your sense of taste
Makes saliva and your tears, muscles move your face
Vestibulocochlear, sense from inner ear
The vestibule's for balancing, the 8th nerve lets you hear
Glossopharyngeal, mixed nerve #9
Impulses come from the throat, swallowing real fine
Mixed Vagus #10, organs kept in check
The Spinal Accessory, 11 moves back, neck
Hypoglossal, 12, muscles move the tongue
Cranial nerves 1 to 12, the song has now been sung

This one is simpler than the first song mentioned before, but it includes less content than that one. Students can choose the most suitable song according to their learning situation and memory ability.

This condition not only exists in the cranial nerves, but also have a lot of memory songs in other medical learning like the HEART ANATOMY SONG, THE MUSCLES SONG, the SKELETON BONES SONG and so on.

MUSIC MNEMONICS IN PHARMACOLOGY

However, in the study of pharmacology, few students realize that music mnemonics is a good way to learn. Students generally report that pharmacology courses are difficult, some students say that the name of the drug is too complicated to remember, otherwise, the names of some drugs are very similar, which makes it easy for students to get confused when memorizing them.

For many students, they learn pharmacology mostly by rote memorization, and don't realize that there are other ways to learn. Their mastery of pharmacology knowledge is not satisfactory in terms of GPA, and the lack of pharmacology basic knowledge in clinical practice and future research also brings them a great deal of adverse influence.

Therefore, it is very important for students, educational institutions and educators to find a suitable mnemonic method.

So, it is believed that if someone tell them there's an easy and efficient way to learn pharmacology, they'd be happy to try it.

So, how to use musical mnemonics? It mainly includes two aspects:

1. Make up songs or fill in lyrics.

By using witty acronyms, wordplay, and memorable poems to compose memory songs. Many teachers in the teaching of the application of this method, the preparation of "Pinyin alphabet song", "English alphabet song", "chemical elements song" to teach students to sing, received amazing effect. The music department of Southwest Normal University in Sichuan province has compiled a tape called "Knowledge Lyrics and Songs Collection" for students to memorize a lot of knowledge through singing.

What's more, we all know that the difficulty of memorizing meaningless words or words is much greater than the speed of memorizing a list of meaningful words or words. So when we memorize information, we first have to do two steps:

1. Is there any connection between the knowledge I want to memorize and the previous knowledge? What is the connection?
2. Whether the knowledge I want to memorize is self-contained, and what is the relationship between the knowledge points?

Once you've done these two steps, you're ready to try mnemonics. Which means connecting the knowledge points that need to be memorized in the lyrics would be better.

Let's try this method.

For example, when we want to memorize the Classes of Antibiotics and Pharmacodynamic Profile of this table below(figure 2):

We can easily find in this table, the Pharmacodynamic Profile of Antibiotics are about three class: Concentration-dependent, Time-dependent, and limited data.

So we can mark Concentration-dependent as C, Time-dependent as T, and the last special one can memorize alone. If you think it's not enough to make a song of these information, you can add other knowledge as you want. Then using a suitable song that you are familiar with to fill in the new words. Sometimes you don't need to fill in a whole melody, just use the ones you know best and can repeat them multiple times.

Figure 2. Pharmacodynamics of common antibiotic classes

Pharmacodynamics of common antibiotic classes (5,6)

Antibiotic Class	Pharmacodynamic Profile	Pharmacodynamic Parameter to Optimize
Aminoglycosides	Concentration-dependent	Peak:MIC
Penicillins	Time-dependent	Time>MIC
Cephalosporins	Time-dependent	Time>MIC
Carbapenems	Time-dependent	Time>MIC
Vancomycin	Time-dependent	AUC:MIC
Lipopeptides	Concentration-dependent	AUC:MIC; peak:MIC
Oxazolidinones	Time-dependent	AUC:MIC
Lipoglycopeptides	Concentration-dependent	AUC:MIC
Fluoroquinolones	Concentration dependent	AUC:MIC
Macrolides	Time-dependent	AUC:MIC
Sulfamethoxazole-trimethoprim	Limited data (65)	Limited data (65)

Here are my songs based on this table (with melody of Sea Shanty Medley):

There once were some medicines that need to see.
And the name oh the medicines were the antibiotics
the Pharmacodynamic Profile fall into two categories
one is T type and the other is the C
First T is the Penicillins
Earliest against staphylococcus and streptococcus
Second T is the Cephalosporins
Gram-positive bacteria againsted by it first
Third T is the Carbapenems
Used in the treatment of severe bacterial infections
Forth T is the Vancomycin
A glycopeptide antibiotic used to treat bacterial infections
Fifth T is the Oxazolidinones
Against Gram-positive bacteria is a synthetic drugs
The last T is the Macrolides
Now used as immunosuppressant drugs
Now we come to the type C of those antibiotics
Which number is less
First we get the Aminoglycosides

Gram-negative antibacterial medications that inhibit protein synthesis
Then we have the Lipopeptides
US FDA approved for complicated skin and skin structure infections
Also same to the Lipoglycopeptides
The last C is the Fluoroquinolones
taken by mouth, some can be given intravenously or as ear or eye drops.

Students can creative their own songs to remember, these memory points are also more impressive when we try to fill out the lyrics.

2. Often sing relaxed and happy music.

While studying or memorizing, play your favorite music at a suitable volume. It helps to learn easily. If it doesn't feel like it,You can slowly develop interest, if you don't feel comfortable, you don't have to force.

Such as Christmas songs, Spring Festival songs, which are very lively and cheerful, and also also very brainwashing. If you can fill in the pharmacology with these melodies, you always can sing them unconsciously, which is very useful for your relaxing study of pharmacology.

CONCLUSION AND FUTURE PROSPECTS

We can speculate that students and teachers are indeed happy to use music amnesia in conjunction with pharmacology and could easily do. Users made it clear that teachers' sharing mnemonic methods with students played an important role, and some of them showed that the songs are valuable when preparing for exams.

Everyone has a different personality and experience, which is reflected in their different views on medical memory songs. As for my personal experience with musical memory, I can definitely say that creative medical memory songs helped me recall information during my study of pharmacology. But the problem with the sample is that the sample data is few, therefore, a large number of experiments are needed to find ways to make students use music memorization correctly and extensively.

REFERENCES

Aloia, D. (2016). Medical Rhymes. *Nyamhistorymed*. https://nyamcenterforhistory.org/2016/04/21/medical-rhymes/

Cirigliano, M. M. (2013). Musical mnemonics in health science: A first look. *Medical Teacher, 35*(3), e1020–e1026. https://doi.org/10.3109/0142159X.2012.733042

Cree, W. J. (1944) In memoriam: Hugo Erichsen M.D. *Detroit Medical News, 36*(12), 9.

Erichsen, H., St. Louis, M. O., & Chambers, J. H. (1884) Medical Rhymes.

Eyler, R. F., & Shvets, K. (2019). Clinical Pharmacology of Antibiotics. *Clinical Journal of the American Society of Nephrology; CJASN, 14*(7), 1080–1090. https://doi.org/10.2215/CJN.08140718

Ezmed. (2022, January 20). *Cranial Nerves MADE EASY: Mnemonic & Tricks for Their Names & Function.* [Video] YouTube. https://www.youtube.com/watch?v=fELPJIjC7E4

Glenn Schellenberg, E. (2011). Music lessons, emotional intelligence, and IQ. *Music Perception, 29*(2), 185–194.

Hargreaves, D. J., MacDonald, R., & Miell, D. (2018). Musical identities mediate musical development. *Music and music education in people's lives, 1*, 124-142.

Hickok, G., Buchsbaum, B., Humphries, C., & Muftuler, T. (2003). Auditory–motor interaction revealed by fMRI: Speech, music, and working memory in area Spt. *Journal of Cognitive Neuroscience, 15*(5), 673–682.

Neural academy. (2020, February 7). *CRANIAL NERVES SONG*. [Video] YouTube. https://www.youtube.com/watch?v=Omair2f46IY&t=29s

Salazar, R. (2000). How to increase your medical memory. *BMJ (Clinical Research Ed.), 321*, 0007245. doi:10.1136bmj.0007245

Saravolatz, L. D., & Stein, G. E. (2015). Oritavancin: A Long-Half-Life Lipoglycopeptide. *Nephrology, Dialysis, Transplantation, 61*(4), 627–632. https://doi.org/10.1093/cid/civ311

Schmid, K. L. (2021). Fluoroquinolones are a potent form of chemotherapy. *Clinical & Experimental Optometry, 104*(3), 412–416. https://doi.org/10.1111/cxo.13102

Scrubssurgicalsoc. (2012, January 30). *The Twelve Cranial Nerves of Christmas.* [Video] YouTube. https://www.youtube.com/watch?v=PcQyJR4dGxc&t=80s

Scrubssurgicalsoc. (2013, September 7). *Learnthroughsong*. [Video] YouTube. https://www.youtube.com/watch?v=0lbwshg_Kj4

Simmons-Stern, N. R., Budson, A. E., & Ally, B. A. (2010). Music as a memory enhancer in patients with Alzheimer's disease. *Neuropsychologia*, *48*(10), 3164–3167. https://doi.org/10.1016/j.neuropsychologia.2010.04.033

Strickland, A.. (2022). What Music Reveals about Our Minds. *CNN Health*. https://www.cnn.com/2022/04/07/health/music-brain-wellness-scn

Thaut, M. H., Peterson, D. A., McIntosh, G. C., & Hoemberg, V. (2014). Music mnemonics aid Verbal Memory and Induce Learning - Related Brain Plasticity in Multiple Sclerosis. *Frontiers in Human Neuroscience*, *8*, 395. https://doi.org/10.3389/fnhum.2014.00395

Chapter 8
Teaching Pharmacology to Complementary and Alternative Medicine Students

Muhammad Asif
The Islamia University of Bahawalpur, Pakistan

Ahsan Zahid
The Islamia University of Bahawalpur, Pakistan

Rabia Zahid
The Islamia University of Bahawalpur, Pakistan

Uzma Bashir
The Islamia University of Bahawalpur, Pakistan

Misbah Firdous
The Islamia University of Bahawalpur, Pakistan

Muhammad Hasnain
https://orcid.org/0000-0003-1705-7751
The Islamia University of Bahawalpur, Pakistan

EXECUTIVE SUMMARY

The field of complementary medicine (CM) is still thriving in several nations. A rise in enrollment at CM educational establishments in both public and private tertiary sectors has indeed been tightly linked to the global popularity of CM. This work presents the very first critical analysis of relevant research analyzing CM education research in direct response to this significant gap. 18 publications out of the 9496 that were found matched the study's criteria for inclusion (English language, kind of CM professionals' education), and they focused on four main problems: CM educational offerings and provision; the development of educational competencies to develop clinical skills and standards; the application of new educational theory, methods and technology in CM; and future challenges facing CM education. This

DOI: 10.4018/978-1-6684-7828-8.ch008

critical integrative review highlights two key issues of interest and significance for CM educational institutions, CM regulators, and researchers, and points to a number of significant gaps in this area of research.

INTRODUCTION

Alternative therapies (CM) are a variety of treatments, products, and strategies for health and ailment that are not generally associated with the medical world or medical coursework. CM is practiced, adopted, and economically viable in many nations, and at the same time, enrollment in CM educational facilities has continued to increase. Organizations offering CM education, including complementary therapies, nutritive medicine, homeopathy, acupuncture, massage therapy, and herbal medicine, are spread throughout the governmental and private tourist sector in many countries, particularly Australia, the United States, the United Kingdom, and Asia. With continuing professional education, educational standards, levels of fundamental biomedicine, and greater levels of certifications appearing in recent years, the professionalization of the CM education sector looks to be increasing, (Gray, 2022).

Academic institutions encounter a plethora of difficulties. This would include enabling CM students to implement primarily conventional concepts and ideas as clinical staff in a modern healthcare environment. Interactive training in inter-professional care presents another problem because the emphasis throughout education is frequently on acquiring a traditional methodology or ideology. Provision of education on scientific proof health coverage presents significant challenges because schooling often focuses on learning and applying conventional proof, which is described in this context as the knowledge that has been passed from father oral administration over many generations after generation and has a lengthy and consistent background of use and is well recorded in pharmacopeias like pharmacopeia and other messages. This would be relevant in a sector with 700 Randomized published studies as well as one that values conventional proof and expertise highly, (Akoko, 2020). Problems include obtaining funds for and offering instruction relevant to CM techniques that are viewed as not being credible in typical educational settings, helping non-traditional learners, and giving details on patient-centered treatment. Additionally, issues with advancements in technology and their impacts on students, instructors, and organizations are still presenting themselves to leadership in academia both inside and outside of CM. For academic institutions, student organizations, and regulations, new innovations in medicine, such as e-health/telehealth, and a rise in attention in the philosophy and instructional methods of online learning in general pose obstacles. In addition to these more regular educational difficulties, current studies and discussions in health promotion have focused on academic opposition to shifting, the technological gap among students and teachers, and virtual preparation for studying. The use of the internet by university students in their academic and personal lives is growing, and innovative learning and teaching in universities are now almost taken for granted in several university courses, (Binks, 2021). This trend goes well beyond studies of CM specifically. Future studies are needed on this subject because CM education is not exempt from such situations.

There have been several studies that investigated the prevalence and perspectives on CM in traditional medical education, biological development, midwives, pharmacology, and hospital coaching, which is in complete contradiction to the literature on CM specialist learning, (). Ironically, a large portion of studies on CM education focuses on its significance and approval process in the nursing curriculum, on the integration of complementary therapies into allied health academic activities, on educating doctors concerning their clients' CM, or on overcoming challenges to implementing transformation in how science is delivered in healthcare.

In order to just provide scientific proof, and coordinated, and multi-professional concern inside this larger health service, the expanding CM workplace requires practice. Building the evidential basis on this subject will benefit the CM sector as well as potentially offer additional insight for health/medical education more generally. Considering the existing environment is essential to building a strong research basis on this subject (Vamos, 2020). Sadly, there hasn't yet been a thorough analysis of peer-reviewed studies on CM education. This report introduces the first comprehensive evaluation of recent papers exploring a variety of crucial issues throughout the CM area of education in spontaneous reaction to this major research deficit.

CM EDUCATION PROVISION

Three publications that gave a straightforward overview of educational offerings in a CM area were found in the study. In one research, the Australian curriculum for alternative medicine and homeopathy was examined. On websites on which they were available, recognized homeopathic curriculum formats and topic area summaries were checked. In certain cases, brief carry conversations were also done. This research examined at how much of the syllabus is decided to devote to clinical experience and biomedical science. It was discovered that ordinary, alternative medicine programs expend 45.9 percent of about their syllabus to health research, while college naturopathy programs devote 26.2% and non-university alternative therapies programs 23.1% respectively (Holst & Health, 2020). Other studies investigated the prevalence of certified comprehensive and section programs as well as certified and non-accredited programs throughout European and commented on the range of training options available in homeopathy. In such typically modest schools, this inter-study of 85 homeopathy academic institutions revealed a mean of 47 enrolled students and 142 graduates. Courses lasting an average of 3.6 years section. In the research institutes, there were 992 total average instruction hours, 555 of which were spent on didactic homeopathy study and the remaining hours on medical experience. The statistics, experience, difficulties, and goals of homeopathic students, teachers, and educational leaders in North America were the subject of a related 2009 study. The study included three independent questionnaires with 40 questions each, with a success rate of 91.5%, that were aimed at homeopathy students, teachers, and school directors (Vassan, 2019). There were discovered to be 29 homeopathic schools in the US, with 250 teachers educating 1080 students. The length of the programs varied greatly; Less than half of the courses, which typically lasted 3.6 years part-time, were completed, but even so, the usual program's (670 hours) length just met the requirements for homeopathic certification. Instructors of homeopathy are typically older than either of the students and practitioners of the discipline. Students are 54.3 years old on the mean. Although women comprise the majority of professionals (75%) and students (90%) respectively, males are substantially more prevalent as teachers (43.5%) and school administrators (45%) (Barreira et al., 2018). Homeopathic school directors are largely (85%) Caucasian, like homeopathy students, practitioners, and teachers. The fact that homeopathic learning in the United States has essentially stagnated over the past ten years was a significant finding. Despite the fact that many new schools have opened, many more have shut.

THE DEVELOPMENT OF EDUCATIONAL COMPETENCIES TO DEVELOP CLINICAL SKILLS AND STANDARDS

Eight publications from the study concentrated on enhancing clinical competence and education in CM. In one study, 43 schooling providers for naturopathy and European traditional remedies in Australia were surveyed for their findings. The results showed that there were significant differences in educational standards, along with inappropriate differences in grant types, course contents, medicinal and pharmaceutical, course duration, and review course. According to this analysis, a bachelor's degree is required for the greater coordination of herbal remedies with conventional medicine. These eight papers all had as their main subject the development or application of learning abilities. When referring to competencies and qualifications, these criteria provide an organized list of capabilities and skills needed. Interview sessions with 17 instructors from various schools in 10 different European nations were done as part of a research project that focused on the expertise, information, qualities, and competencies of homeopaths and the implementation of homeopathy education. In order to establish classifications and characteristics of educational needs and theoretical constructs as well as to explain interaction and social processes, this qualitative research used continuous comparisons and analyses. It revealed to educators that a qualified homeopath is a practitioner who is capable of helping physicians in the best approach. It was discovered that the ability has to be patient-centered for both students and homeopaths, as well as program administrators and instructors (Taff, 2020). The contrast of frequent academic development in and application of both Western and CM diagnostic approaches, it was observed in an Australian study that CM practitioners lacked confidence in their ability to recognize clients who needed to be sent to licensed health professionals.

The combination of alternative and traditional medicines in CM schools, as well as the training of certain components of professional effective communication, were the topic of two papers that were found. The communication between conventional physicians and CM practitioners was discussed by 62 students in Israel using a pre-course "semi-structured questionnaire" and questionnaires following an education program (Gray, 2022). This study discovered that when they employed critical thinking, patient-centered care, and other CM strategies, CM practitioners were more prepared to interact with traditional healthcare care professionals. and interacting was stressed throughout their university education. In fact, results from 28 administrators of colleges of CM were reported by a Canadian study. According to the authors, communication with conventional care providers requires that students be able to comprehend research outcomes, rely on elevated scientific, and participate in continuous education.

Three studies focused on the necessity for schools to develop research literacy and evidence-based practice skills. One investigation that looked at the views of 202 faculty academics in an Australian CM college regarding research and scholarly activities revealed low trust in collecting data. In this Australian study, people feel that research was crucial to achieving their goals both professionally and personally (86.0%), but they were less confident in their ability to conduct studies (56.5%) (McLean et al., 2019). Even though the respondents' trust in their own capacity to create research papers was lower (52.9%), they still regarded the value of publishing of study to their own professional aspirations to be very high (80.0%). The study done in the US looked at the methods used by 9 CM colleges to build evidence-based skills and knowledge with the goal of teaching professors and students how to critically analyze research and use it to improve clinical practice. According to this research, academic institutions adopted tactics that have been thought to be essential for success while creating the framework for their educational programs, such as creating them diverse and distinctive to their specific organizational requirements. These techniques were discovered to be effective in different CM and non-CM academic institutions where executives were thinking about integrating research literacy and EBP competencies into their curricula when used in conjunction with preexisting instructional methodologies. The most effective method for educating faculty in scientific proof medicine and research literacy was determined to be mandatory training and seminars. Finally, one evaluated paper discussed the institutional teaching methodologies and educational competencies that had been created and put into place at all nine R25-funded CM institutions in the US to improve research literacy (Edwards, 2023). This study discovered that although each establishment developed strategies that suited all its scientific temper, the core principles were common to all, indicating that it was crucial to develop evidence-informed skills and knowledge to support both instructors and students as they main investigation critically and apply it to advise their medical practice. The tactics used by these universities included the requirement that faculty members be open to acquiring and teaching EBM abilities, and that core curriculum be suitable to reinforcing EBM competencies utilizing spiral instructional methods.

Cm Implementation of Current and Emerging Educational Philosophy, Methodologies, And Technology

Six papers that were part of the evaluation shed light just on evolving role of a trainer/lecturer in instructional and clinical subject areas, the application of old and new learning philosophy, the use of issues in the context of CM curriculum content in Bachelor of Science and medical college programs, as well as the expanding need for learning technologies. Various education initiatives evaluating novel teaching techniques were implemented inside an Ayurvedic curriculum in one research. An integrative module on cardiovascular physiology, case-stimulated knowledge, and discussions in small groups in the schoolroom was the prospect of improvement that has been assessed. The results indicated that the innovation of verifiable interdisciplinary teaching techniques is feasible in the sense of Ayurveda education(Edwards, 2023) The application of a goal-formalized clinical assessment (OSCE) concept and a patient-centered training strategy in under traditional Chinese medicine (TCM) physician schooling in one Taiwanese medical school, on the other hand, was discovered to be a successful instructional invasion that improved the standard of TCM practices by evaluating, attempting to teach, and certifying TCM clinical qualifications. TCM internal medicine, TCM gynecology, TCM pediatrics, TCM dietetics, acupuncture, TCM orthopedics, and traumatology were among the training program subjects in this research.

Figure 1. Existing and new educational theory, methods and technology in CM

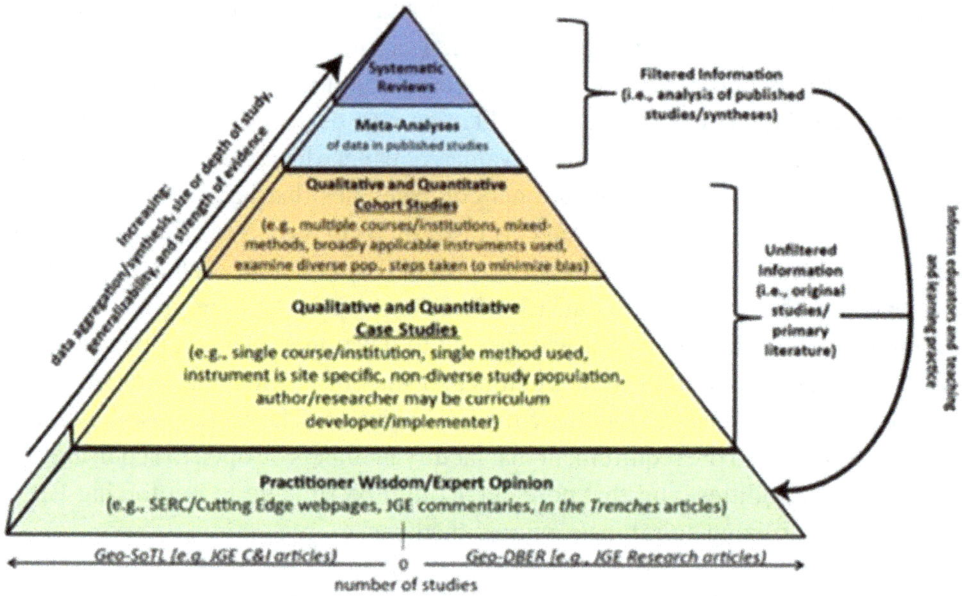

In order to understand how former and current educators of four-year natural medicine degree programs in Australia engage with clinical teaching materials as well as their perceptions and beliefs toward teaching materials in naturopathic learning, Wardle's 2014 study used focus groups with these students. According to this survey, natural medicine students want the current curricula to emphasize evidence-based methods and knowledge that both supports and critiques conventional naturopath practices(Steel, 2019). These scholars were mostly apathetic toward new teaching techniques and preferred that they evolve naturally from hard copies rather than suddenly and violently diverge from them. The findings of an inter-research survey from 27-item questionnaires provided to 1-4-year Orthopedic medical graduates in the United States CM students' effective teaching methods are frequently focused on levels of computing knowledge and experience, with their current use of computers as a teaching resource, and behaviors concerning the function of computer systems in medical training. Wiki pages, webcasts, and synchronous audio-based online interactions are just a few of the innovations that one research project of natural medicine faculty found was well-accepted for use in effective learning. The study was based on interview sessions with faculty carried out in the Australian education sector. Acupuncture, chiropractic, and massage therapy professors, on the other hand, were found in a different US study to be unaware of the benefits of internet-based learning and the components of effective online courses computing knowledge and experience, with their current use of computers as a teaching resource, and behaviors concerning the function of computer systems in medical training (Hwang, 2020).

PRIORITIES AND POSSIBILITIES FOR EXPLORATION

Wiki pages, webcasts, and concurrent audio-based online interactions are just a few of the innovations that one research project of natural medicine faculty found was well-accepted for use in effective learning. The study was based on interview sessions with faculty carried out in the Australian education sector. Acupuncture, chiropractic, and massage therapy professors, on the other hand, were found in a different US study to be unaware of the benefits of internet-based teaching and the components of effective online courses.

Understanding CM students' and teachers' physical location, student enrollment trends, instructional methods, scale, and scope, as well as global parallels and contrasts, is urgently necessary. This is crucial because of the largely undeveloped and possibly identification and characterization of CM academic institutions, as well as their similarities and distinctions with other medical services academic achievement (nursing, pharmacy), the prospective volume of the CM education sector, and the percentage of graduates accessing CM professions. In addition, a more thorough investigation of staff perspectives toward changes and technology, as well as faculty demography, psychographic segmentation, and beliefs, is required in CM colleges. Going forward, it will be important to comprehend how shifting educational trends relate to CM, whether CM educational settings are distinctive due to their particular student populations, the distinction between training CM practitioners and teaching others how to use CM, the vastly diverse landscape of CM education provision around the world, and the extent to which CM education systems are effected by broadening developments occurring globally (Mense, 2018). Massive Online Courses (MOOCs), classroom methods, constructivist education concepts, and the adoption of problem-based learning are just a few of the changes that are occurring in learning internationally. This highlights the way forward for CM educational psychology. Such a review of CM training must also take into account local laws and subtleties, as well as the educational system's variety in terms of culture. It is also necessary to have a deeper understanding of how CM training is influenced by medical services education, the extent to which research and evidence from health services education may be scaled to CM education, and how the fundamental sciences are taught at CM institutions. Colleges might find it useful to investigate methods for training professors in subjects like e-learning technology, research competence, and scientific proof practice skills, as well as students in subjects like data literacy and health education. For this, adopters and change leaders are required in addition to academic and administration champions. There is still much to learn about the vast array of education opportunities offered by CM globally. working to promote CM-related coursework in postsecondary learning generally, such as meditation or completed, as well as the variety of award choices with courses presently offered at the graduation level, the connection among preconditions, the composition of the program, and the bachelor's degree outcome, as well as routes Those basic education programs, entrance requirements, and background knowledge before CM training could raise professional standards, publishing output, and scientifically knowledge(Wong, 2022). The economic motivations of for-profit private equity educational institutions in the CM profession must also be better understood.

Figure 2. Domains of complementary medicine and alternative medicine

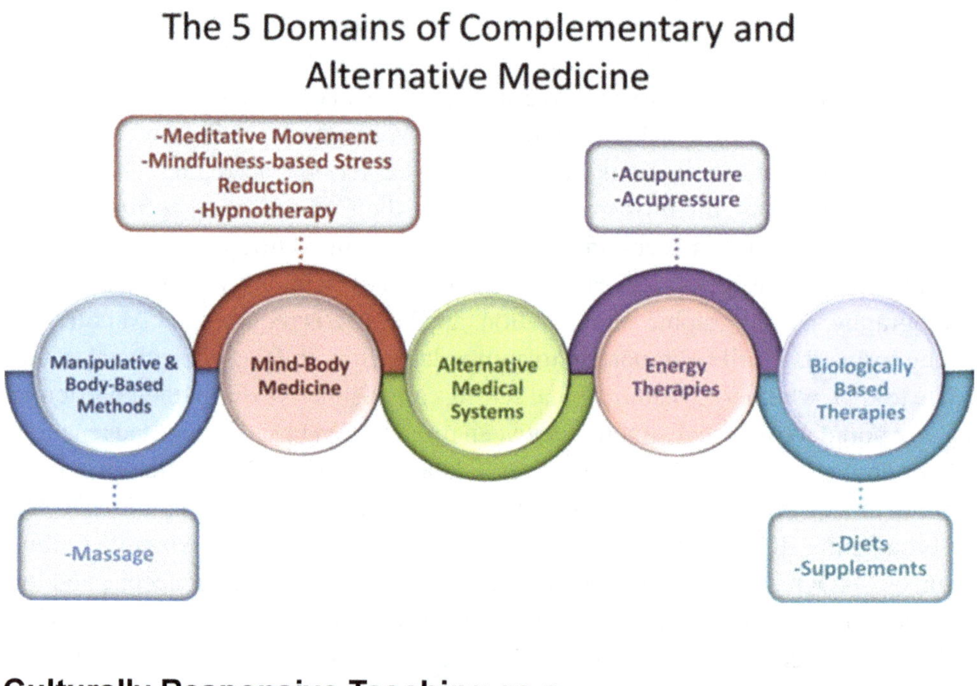

Culturally Responsive Teaching as a Bridge Between Frameworks

Working to promote CM-related coursework in postsecondary learning generally, such as meditation or completed, in addition to the variety of award choices with course work presently offered at the graduation level, the connection among preconditions, the composition of the program, and the bachelor's degree outcome, as well as routes Those basic education programs, entrance exams, and background knowledge before CM training could raise standards of practice, publishing output, and scientifically knowledge. The economic motivations of for-profit private equity academic institutions in the CM profession must also be better understood (Bos et al., 2020). It might be a workable method for applying a mixed strategy to incorporate diverse cultures into courses. Since it can handle culturally diverse training for aspiring pharmacists, enhance learning settings, and perhaps even lessen achievement gaps, introducing culturally responsive instruction as a methodology has appeal. Creating cultural exchange socialization, using a variety of teaching techniques to meet students' needs, becoming aware of the ethnic diversity in the classroom, developing culturally significant curricula, and exhibiting cultural sympathy are the five key components of using culturally responsive teaching in an educational environment. The first two facets of culturally responsive teaching have been exemplified and promoted by culturally diverse instructors in teaching and learning, as seen by the abundance of possibilities available to learners. An environment that encourages cultural socialization, for instance, has been developed by pharmacist educators who include components of community engagement, service-learning, or global health outreach in their courses. Additionally, teachers that use case studies, group activities, technologies, and other teaching techniques to involve students in class have given students a variety of ways to study. These last three components, though, require more investigation. The third component—learning the cultural diversity of the class—seems to be the most challenging for pharmacy instructors to accomplish, according to research. For instance, a study evaluating health care educators, including pharmacist educators, discovered that 70% of respondents said they lacked the expertise necessary to teach people from different cultural backgrounds (Secchi, 2022). Worse than that, offensive remarks done by professors can harm learning settings and uphold the demeaning habit of not respecting in a way that goes further than the classroom. The majority of activities in university education have been focused on "yet another" capacity-building workshop or online program. However, the effects of such remarks and interactions highlight how crucial and necessary it is to invest heavily in professional learning.

Ethnic Variety and Faculty from the Faculty's Vision

Evaluating faculty perceptions of diverse cultures is the first step in educating faculty to become culturally responsive educators from the viewpoint of effectiveness. Faculty viewpoints might range from an individualist viewpoint to one that is deficient-oriented. According to a deficit-oriented viewpoint, learners' development and ability are related. For instance, some educators can think that, due to their upbringing, kids from different cultural backgrounds are prevented from meeting particular requirements (Tomasik et al., 2021). More particular, a teacher who employs a deficit-oriented strategy may anticipate strong performance from

Asian American children because their culture values academic brilliance. This strategy is patently incorrect and will not help student pharmacies grow in terms of the four cultural humility ideals or exemplify the five components of culturally appropriate instruction. In contrast side, the institutional technique works to lower organizational barriers to level the playing field for learners. Providing pupils with regular objectives and exposure to a challenging, well-taught course are only two examples of academic resources and opportunities. We currently use a systemic method to teach pharmacy students about cultural diversity. Everywhere in our Academies, student pharmacists have the chance to experience cultural diversity through programs on culture, service learning, and global health projects (Chan, 2018). As a result, a teacher using a systemic approach might make the most of the resources allocated to cultural diversity training and demand a certain degree of proficiency from each student. Even though this strategy may include some parts of cultural humility, tangible results, such as the decrease in health inequities we previously highlighted, have not yet been attained. As an alternative, educators who take an emancipatory stance value and promote student variety. An instructor that favors an emergent method would motivate learners to first consider how their culture has affected their well-being before guiding a topic utilizing high school senior experiences within the context of pharmacy education. An effective emancipatory strategy emphasizes the above-noted four major integrity tenets: self-reflection/self-criticism, teaching from a patient, developing a patient-practitioner collaboration, and accepting a lifetime process. This method also equips teachers to use culturally sensitive methods of instruction within the classroom. It would be necessary for faculty to embrace and adopt an emancipatory approach to education across the curriculum in order to move in this direction (Louis & King, 2022). To address our current diversity concerns in a way that is relevant to the demographic changes in the US, developing strong continuous training for academics is essential. Isolated sessions have not shown indications of affecting specific student performance or indicating improvements in educators' methods. Rather, "best practices" must be included in clearly defined faculty development programs. One of the finest methods for faculty development is called "shadow coaching," inside which mentorship assists individual teachers by routinely giving feedback in the classroom and encouraging teachers to reflect and critically examine their objectives, methods of instruction, and evaluation methods. Along with regular meetings, shadow teaching also entails groups of mentors and mentees reflecting collectively on their achievements and coming up with answers to issues that arise in their particular courses (Dennen, 2022). It is deliberate and focused joining after continuing faculty peer observations that ensure faculty use successful teaching methodologies. However, avoid misdating crucial components since this could lead to unexpected changes in culturally relevant education. Academic staff who have pursued advanced training in learning and completed courses via colleges or departments of education toward certificates or degrees are potential sources of supervisors qualified to offer to shadow tutoring at a school or institution of pharmacists. Pharmacy instructors might make requests for mentoring who have received training in culturally sensitive mentoring from university-wide organizations such as centers for education and learning. From the standpoint of evaluation, key tools to support culturally responsive practices for academic staff include the Learning Multicultural Attitude Survey, the Multicultural Teaching Competency Scale, and culturally responsive teaching rubrics like those created by Kea and Trent.

ABBREVIATIONS

Table 1.

Complementary Medicine	CM
Mixed Methods Appraisal Too	MOOC
Traditional Chinese medicine	TCM
Evidence-based practice	EBP

CONCLUSION

Finally, we recognized some of the issues facing the Australian naturopathic profession in our assessment, including naturopathic education, the changing makeup of pharmaceutical students, homeopathic students' demands, and the rising conflict among conventional and scientific proof. In this research, which involved semi-structured discussions to 20 traditional healers, it was discovered that people who participated explained a phenomenon in which they sponsored the learning of more biological sciences in natural medicine teaching while also criticizing the pattern for modern natural medicine schooling to "become more scientific"—a trend they attributed to their desire for the discipline to be "acknowledged in the tertiary education sector." Others suggested that such progress might be carried out at the expense of the institution's foundational principles. The researchers concluded that maintaining ethical and efficient therapeutic interventions required the continuous creation of minimal professional standards and instruction that value conventional homeopathic concepts and concepts, together with the establishment of suitable regulatory mechanisms.

Conflict Of Interest

No conflict of interest was found among the authors.

ACKNOWLEDGEMENT

We would like to thank Prof. Dr. Naveed Akhter for his knowledge and support across all areas of our research as well as for his cooperation in preparing the chapter.

REFERENCES

Akoko, J. (2020). Serological and molecular evidence of Brucella species in the rapidly growing pig sector in Kenya. *BioMed Central, 16*(1), 1-7.

Barreira, P., Basilico, M., & Bolotnyy, V. J. H. U. (2018). Graduate student mental health: Lessons from American economics departments. *NIH.*

Binks, A.P., (2021). Changing medical education, overnight: the curricular response to COVID-19 of nine medical schools. *NIH, 33*(3), p. 334-342.

Bos, A., Kruse, F.M., & Jeurissen, P. (2020). *For-profit nursing homes in the Netherlands: what factors explain their rise? NIH,* (4), p. 431-443.

Chan, W. (2018). President's Whitepaper Project: Global Literacy at the University of Maryland, Baltimore. University of Maryland.

Dennen, V.P. (2022). Supporting new online instructors and engaging remote learners during COVID-19: a distributed team teaching approach. *NIH, 54*(sup1), S182-S202.

Edwards, N. (2023). *Research Education Program for Underrepresented Minority Students: Students' Perception of Academic Enrichment and Research Activities.* NIH.

Gayatri, D. (2021). Quality of life of cancer patients at palliative care units in developing countries: systematic review of the published literature. *NIH, 30*(2), 315-343.

Gray, A.C. (2022). *An examination of the prevalence, impact, experiences and perceptions of learning and health technologies on students, academics and educational leaders in complementary medicine education institutions: A mixed method study of two institutions, one in Australia and one in the US.* University of Technology Sydney.

Holst, J. & Health, P. (2020). Increasing rural recruitment and retention through rural exposure during undergraduate training: an integrative review. *NIH, 17*(17): p. 6423.

Hwang, G.-J. (2020). *Vision, challenges, roles and research issues of Artificial Intelligence in Education*. Elsevier. doi:10.1016/j.caeai.2020.100001

Louis, V.N. & King, N. (2022). Emancipating STEM education through abolitionist teaching: A research-practice partnership to support virtual microteaching experiences. *NIH, 33*(2), 206-226.

McLean, S.A., Caldwell, B., & Roberton, M. (2019). *Reach Out and Recover: Intentions to seek treatment in individuals using online support for eating disorders*. NIH.

Mense, E.G. (2018). The development of global higher education in a world of transformation. *NIH, 2*(3), 47.

Secchi, A. (2022). Medication management in m inority, a sian and b lack ethnic older people in the United Kingdom: a mixed-studies systematic review. *NIH, 47*(9): p. 1322-1336.

Steel, A. (2019). *The role and influence of traditional and scientific knowledge in naturopathic education: a qualitative study. NIH, 25*(2), p. 196-201.

Taff, S. D. (2020). *Educator's guide for addressing cultural awareness, humility, and dexterity in occupational therapy curricula*. Washington University.

Tomasik, M.J., Helbling, L.A. & Moser, U. (2021). Educational gains of in-person vs. distance learning in primary and secondary schools: A natural experiment during the COVID-19 pandemic school closures in Switzerland. *NIH, 56*(4), 566-576.

Vamos, S. (2020). *Making a case for "Education for health literacy": An international perspective. MDPI, 17*(4), 1436.

Vassan, J. G. (2019). *Perceptions of Homoeopathic Practitioners Regarding Continuing Professional Development (CPD) in South Africa*. University of Johannesburg.

Wong, J.T. (2022). *A learning experience design approach to online professional development for teaching science through the arts: Evaluation of teacher content knowledge, self-efficacy and STEAM perceptions,* p. 1-31. NIH.

Chapter 9
Pharmacological Evidence on Drug-Herbal Interactions on the Human Body:
Drug-herb Interactions Between Cardiovascular Drugs and Chinese Herbs

Tan Chia Hui
Xiamen University Malaysia, Malaysia

Wen Wen Lee
Xiamen University Malaysia, Malaysia

Jian Xin Chu
Xiamen University Malaysia, Malaysia

Ching Hua Ng
Xiamen University Malaysia, Malaysia

EXECUTIVE SUMMARY

Assessing the potential herb-drug interactions is necessary to ensure clinical safety and to prevent any untoward effects. Studies have identified a variety of adverse effects on herb-drug interactions. Common mechanisms include the modulation of drug-metabolic enzymes, which leads to irreversible impacts. Physicians should constantly double-check if patients see numerous prescribers or visit multiple hospital settings before prescribing drugs to avoid pharmaceutical toxicity. Chinese herbal medicines are an essential part of TCM practice. Thus, the elevation and classification of toxic herb-drug interactions are helpful to ensure the safet usage by practitioners in optimizing the effectiveness of treatment strategies. According to WHO, cardiovascular diseases caused about 17.9 million deaths, accounting for 32% of all global deaths in 2019. This literature review will be focusing on cardiovascular drugs due to the high global mortality rate of cardiovascular diseases.

DOI: 10.4018/978-1-6684-7828-8.ch009

INTRODUCTION

In recent years, a deadly infectious disease known as Coronavirus disease 2019 (COVID-19) had spread rapidly and inflicted a worldwide pandemic. According to the International Journal of Infectious Diseases, more than 1.5 million positive cases were recorded globally about four months after SARS-CoV-2 infection had been first discovered in China (Shah et al., 2020). It is different from the SARS outbreak in 2003. Traditional Chinese Medicine (TCM) had displayed efficacy in combating COVID-19 throughout the treatment, with 2000 years of experience in preventing and treating epidemics and plagues. Furthermore, Chinese herbal medicines also have the potential to be one of the therapeutics aids in treating diseases and act as potential materials in maintaining the proper health of humans worldwide.

Based on the Basic and Clinical Pharmacology (14th Edition), a drug may be defined as any substance that brings about a change in biologic function through its chemical actions in the most general sense (Bertram, 2018). A drug is usually used to regulate the biological system in the human body by acting as an agonist or antagonist to the specific receptor. Over time, botanical products sales have increased obviously and more well-known in popularity, especially in the United Stated since National Health Interview Survey had recently revealed that almost 20% of Americans consume this kind of product (Grimstein & Huang, 2018).

However, a crucial issue about the safety quality of Chinese herbal medicines is lacking evidence-based toxicological review on herb-drug interactions. With the high demand for TCM, there will be quite a concern about the quality and safety of using Chinese herbs in therapeutic treatment. A guideline had been given for industry stated by the Food and Drug Administration (FDA), a sponsor should reach an agreement with the appropriate Office of New Drug (OND) review division about the methods they plan to use for arriving at acceptable dose levels in safety pharmacology and toxicity in order to use for safety monitoring during human clinical studies (Food and Drug Administration, 2016).

Therefore, assessing the potential herb-drug interactions is necessary to ensure clinical safety and to prevent any untoward effects. Over the past 40 years, clinical studies have identified a variety of adverse effects on herb-drug interactions. Common mechanisms include modulation of drug-metabolic enzymes, which leads to irreversible impacts. According to the National Law Act, it is imperative for all practitioners to improve their practice standards and monitor patients' health care effectively to provide more quality and safe healthcare services to the public (Kim et al., 2013). Doctors and physicians should constantly double-check if patients see numerous prescribers or visit multiple hospital settings before prescribing drugs to avoid pharmaceutical toxicity. Chinese herbal medicines are an essential part of TCM practice. Thus, the elevation and classification of toxic in herb-drug interactions are helpful to ensure the safety usage by practitioners in optimizing the effectiveness of treatment strategies (Kim et al., 2013). According to World Health Organization (WHO), cardiovascular diseases caused about 17.9 million people died, accounting for 32% of all global deaths in 2019 (World Health Organization, 2021). In the following section, our literature review will be focusing on cardiovascular drugs due to the high global mortality rate of cardiovascular diseases.

LITERATURE REVIEW

Table 1. Reported drug-herb interactions between cardiovascular drugs and Chinese herbs

Drugs	Chinese herbs *(Binomial name)*	Outcome of Drug-herb Interaction	References
Digoxin	Aloe vera (*Aloe barbadensis*)	Potentiates potassium loss and digoxin toxicity risk	(Alissa, 2014)
	Papaya leaf (*Carica papaya* L.)	Inhibits P-gp transport of digoxin	(Lim et al., 2021)
	Chan Su (*Venenum bufonis*)	High interference with digoxin assay	(Tachjian et al., 2010)
	Dan shen (*Salvia miltiorrhiza*)	Increases side effects of digoxin	(Tachjian et al., 2010)
	Eleuthero or Siberian ginseng (*Eleutheroccus senticosus*)	Raises digoxin concentrations in plasma	(Fugh-Berman, 2000)
	Ginkgo (*Ginkgo biloba*)	Increases the AUC and C_{max}	(Parvez et al., 2019)
	Hawthorn (*Crataegus oxyacantha*)	Potentiates in increasing the effects of digoxin on heart contractility	(Beik et al., 2020)
	Liquorice (*Glycyrrhiza glabra*)	Potentiates digoxin toxicity	(Tachjian et al., 2010)
	St John's wort (*Hypericum perforatum*)	Decreases AUC, C_{max}, and C_{trough} of digoxin	(Fugh-Berman, 2000)
Warfarin	Dan shen (*Salvia miltiorrhiza*)	Increases INR, prolonged partial thromboplastin time	(Fugh-Berman, 2000)
	Dong quai (*Angelica sinensis*)	Increases INR and causes bruising	(Fugh-Berman, 2000)
	Garlic (*Allium sativum*)	Increases INR	(Parvez et al., 2019)
	Ginger (*Zingiber officinale*)	Increases bleeding risk	(Tachjian et al., 2010)
	Ginkgo (*Ginkgo biloba*)	Increases bleeding risk	(Tachjian et al., 2010)
	St John's wort (*Hypericum perforatum*)	Decreases INR	(Fugh-Berman, 2000)
Aspirin	Ginkgo (*Ginkgo biloba*)	Increases bleeding risk	(Mohammadi et al., 2020)
	Ginseng (*Panax ginseng*)	Increases bleeding risk	(Mohammadi et al., 2020)
	Evening primrose (*Oenothera biennis*)	Increases effect of aspirin	(Mohammadi et al., 2020)

Abbreviations: P-glycoprotein (P-gp); Digoxin area under the curve (AUC); International normalized ratio (INR); digoxin maximal plasma concentration (C_{max}); digoxin plasma concentration at 24 hours after the previous dosing (C_{trough})

Among cardiovascular diseases, atrial fibrillation (AF) is the most popular arrhythmia encountered in the ICU. AF patients will be given medications for rate or rhythm controls, including nondihydropyridine calcium channel blockers, beta-blockers and digoxin (Bosch, 2018). Throughout the past centuries, digoxin was found to reduce the hospital admission. Digoxin is a cardiac glycoside which is originated from the *Digitalis* (foxglove) plant. It can slow down the heart rate and improve the efficiency of heart in pumping blood (David & Shetty, 2021). However, the drug interactions between digoxin and herbs are important and should be focused as digoxin is a narrow therapeutic index (NTI) drug. NTI drugs are drugs where minor differences in dose or blood concentration may lead to serious therapeutic failures or adverse drug reactions that are life-threatening or result in persistent or significant disability or incapacity (Yu et al., 2015). There are several clinical trials reported that digoxin and herbs possess adverse outcomes of drug-herb interaction.

In 2004, a clinical study about drug-herb interaction between St John's wort (*Hypericum perforatum*) and digoxin was conducted among 96 healthy volunteers. A 7-day loading phase with digoxin was followed by 14 days of comedication and the pharmacokinetics of digoxin were determined before and on the 14th day of comedication. For the result, when high-dose of hyperforin-rich extract LI160 (St. John's wort product that contains a greater amount of hyperforin) is comedicated with digoxin, it reduces digoxin area under the curve from time 0 to 24 hours (AUC_{0-24}) by 24.8% (95% confidence interval [CI], -28.3 to -21.3), reduces C_{max} by 37% (95% CI, -42 to -32), and reduces C_{trough} by 19% (95% CI, -27 to -11). When digoxin is comedicated with 4g of Hypericum powder with comparable hyperforin content, it reduces AUC_{0-24} by 26.6% (95% CI, -37.3 to -15.9), reduces C_{max} by 38% (95% Cl, -48 to -18), and reduces C_{trough} by 19% (95% Cl, -27 to -10). In short, the comedication of St John's wort and digoxin will cause a reduction in the AUC, C_{max}, and C_{trough}. Moreover, the compounds of St John's wort, like hyperforin and hypericin are the mediators of P-glycoprotein induction (MUELLER, 2004).

In a clinical study, eight healthy male volunteers were given St John's Wort extracts for two weeks, which resulted in an 18% decrease of AUC after a single digoxin dose (0.5mg). There is a 1.4- and 1.5-fold increased expressions of duodenal P-glycoprotein/MDR1 and CYP3A4 respectively. As a result, the administration of St John's Wort extracts directly affected the expression of P-glycoprotein/MDR1 and CYP3A4 (hepatic cytochromes P450 3A4) drug transporters in the intestine and the activity of CYP3A4 in the liver as evaluated by the erythromycin breath test (Dürr, 2000).

In 2003, there was another clinical study about the interaction between digoxin and Hawthorn (*Crataegus oxyacantha*). Hawthorn is a herbal supplement that is evaluated for the treatment of heart failure. It is found out that even though both Hawthorn and St John's wort are rich in various flavonols, including rutin, isoquercitrin, quercetin and hyperoside, but Hawthorn only causes mild induction (< 25%) of P-glycoprotein activity. There are no significant differences in AUC,

C_{max}, and C_{trough} values. However, Hawthorn still has the possibility of increasing the digoxin's effect on heart contractility and increasing the heart rate that is contradicted to the digoxin drug effect. Besides, Hawthorn also has the ability to produce endothelium-dependent vasodilation (Tankanow et al., 2003).

The clinical outcomes of herb-drug interaction mainly rely on the nature of the herbs and drug itself. Due to the NTI property of digoxin, its combination with herbal remedies may alter its pharmacokinetics and pharmacodynamics processes after administration, subsequently leading to clinical consequences ranging from mild, severe, or even lethal.

Some herbal medicines share the exact pharmacokinetics mechanism as digoxin. Alteration in either ADME (absorption, distribution, metabolism, and elimination) process can promote pharmacokinetics herb-drug interactions. The efflux transport of digoxin is mediated by P-glycoprotein substrate (P-gp) and metabolized by Cytochrome P450 3A4 (CYP3A4) enzymes. Both are prevalent at the villus tip of enterocytes and hepatocytes, where drug absorption and metabolism occur. As herbal medicines are often administered orally, their concentrations are typically found moderate to high in the gut lumen and liver (Chen et al., 2012), causing potential herb-drug interactions to occur via inhibition or induction of P-gp and CYPs. Modulation of intestinal and hepatic CYPs and P-gp can alter the oral absorption, bioavailability, systemic exposure, biliary or renal clearance, and brain uptake of drugs. For instance, plant products including gum guar (*Cyamopsis tetragonolobus*), acacia gum (*Acacia senegal*), or guggulipid (*Commiphora mukul*) can reduce the absorption of digoxin by binding, trapping, and creating viscous matrices with co-administered digoxin (Izzo, 2012). A minor change in systemic exposure of digoxin might produce a significant shift in its therapeutic efficacy and toxicity outcomes due to the steep dose-response relationship (Chen et al., 2012). Oral administration of St John's wort (*Hypericum perforatum*) by healthy subjects can elevate duodenal P-gp expression by 1.4-fold (Li et al., 2014), primarily due to its reactive component, namely hyperforin (de Lima Toccafondo Vieira & Huang, 2012). In long-term treatment of St John's wort, the plasma level of co-administered digoxin is reduced (Fasinu et al., 2012), thereby exacerbate undesirable conditions such as arrhythmia and hypertension (Suroowan & Mahomoodally, 2015). In some clinical cases, impaired drug efficacy, treatment failure (Davis et al., 2014), or even organ rejection may occur (Parvez & Rishi, 2019). In contrast, some herbal medicines can reduce the clearance and increase the plasma concentrations of digoxin. In this case, consumption of digoxin with Siberian Ginseng (*Eleutheroccus senticosus*) can elevate its serum concentration (Parvez & Rishi, 2019). Consequently, patients are more susceptible to adverse effects and more likely to show toxicity. Because of the shared ADME mechanism, medicinal components having a similar structure to digoxin can be detected in the serum as digoxin and cause the elevation in the level.

Referring to this situation, the primary active constituents of Hawthorn (*Crataegus spp*), namely flavonoids, comprises a polycyclic ring structure similar to digoxin (Dasgupta et al., 2010). This might falsely increase the blood concentration of digoxin, therefore raising the risk of arrhythmias (Liperoti et al., 2017).

Pharmacodynamics herb-drug interaction develops when herbal medicines have either direct additive, synergistic or antagonistic effect on the mechanism of action of digoxin, thereby changing the extent of digoxin response. In most cases of pharmacodynamics herb-drug interaction, synergistic or antagonistic interactions may affect the drug efficacy or lead to organ toxicity. Due to the structural similarity, some herbal compounds may mimic, enhance, or decrease the effects of co-administered digoxin by acting on the same pharmacological targets. The structural similarity allows herbal components to compete with digoxin for binding sites, and it is possible to displace digoxin from the targets of action. Accordingly, some herbal remedies consisting of antagonistic chemicals are likely to lower the efficacy of digoxin and result in therapeutic failure. Direct pharmacologic actions of herbal medicines may antagonize or impair the clinical outcomes without altering blood concentrations (Asher et al., 2017). The intake of danshen (*Salvia miltiorrhiza*) can interfere with digoxin's metabolism (Suroowan & Mahomoodally, 2015), whereas aloe vera (*Aloe barbadensis*), buckthorn (*Rhamnus catartica*), cascara (*Rhamnus purshiani*), licorice (*Glycyrrhiza glabra*), and senna (*Cassia senna*) might cause hypokalaemia (Tsai et al., 2012). As a result of these outcomes, digoxin toxicity may occur and conditions including chronic renal failure, hypomaganesium, hypercalcemia, and hypothyroidism may be observed (Lin et al., 2014)

CONCLUSION

Our literature review highlighted that narrow therapeutic index drugs such as digoxin have more adverse effects or are less effective when used with herbal products. Clinical studies have proven that the combination of digoxin with St John's Wort may impair drug efficacy, treatment failure, or even organ rejection. However, some Chinese herbs have shown no adverse effects when used in conjunction with digoxin. For instance, Echinacea (*Echinacea spp.*), widely used to prevent and treat common infections, such as respiratory tract infections, did not change the pharmacokinetics of digoxin. Discrepancies were shown in various clinical studies for Hawthorn and digoxin interaction. For instance, Hawthorn, used for the treatment of congestive heart failure, showed no effect on the pharmacokinetics of digoxin based on a study in 2003 (Tankanow et al., 2003). A study in 2010 discovered that Hawthorn contains alkaloids structurally like digoxin and may also interfere with digoxin immunoassays (Dasgupta et al., 2010). To date, the interaction between herbs and digoxin remains yet to be elucidated and more clinical studies should be carried out to ensure its safety efficacy before being implemented as a complimentary treatment. A systematic technique and guidelines should be established to address the information gaps in future assessments of interactions between drugs and Chinese herbal prescriptions (Costache et al., 2019). Patients taking digoxin should never practice self-medication to prevent dangerous drug and herbs interaction. Patients are recommended to practice beneficial lifestyle activities such as exercising regularly or having healthy diets instead of concurrently consuming Chinese herbal supplements without professional consultations. As the Chinese saying goes, “It is rather poisonous as a medication”. Lastly, physicians-patients communication should be enhanced, and the former must be ready to investigate the patient’s use of herbs in a non-judgmental approach, which otherwise will only prompt patients to hide valuable information.

REFERENCES

Alissa, E. M. (2014). Medicinal Herbs and Therapeutic Drugs Interactions. *Therapeutic Drug Monitoring*, *36*(4), 413–422. doi:10.1097/FTD.0000000000000035 PMID:24452064

Asher, G. N., Corbett, A. H., & Hawke, R. L. (2017). Common Herbal Dietary Supplement-Drug Interactions. *American Family Physician*, *96*(2), 101–107. PMID:28762712

Beik, A., Joukar, S., & Najafipour, H. (2020). A review on plants and herbal components with antiarrhythmic activities and their interaction with current cardiac drugs. *Journal of Traditional and Complementary Medicine*, *10*(3), 275–287. doi:10.1016/j.jtcme.2020.03.002 PMID:32670823

Bertram, G. K. (2018). *Basic & clinical pharmacology* (14th ed.). McGraw-Hill Education.

Bosch, N. A., Cimini, J., & Walkey, A. J. (2018). Atrial Fibrillation in the ICU. *Chest*, *154*(6), 1424–1434. doi:10.1016/j.chest.2018.03.040 PMID:29627355

Chen, X. W., Sneed, K. B., Pan, S. Y., Cao, C., Kanwar, J. R., Chew, H., & Zhou, S. F. (2012). Herb-drug interactions and mechanistic and clinical considerations. *Current Drug Metabolism*, *13*(5), 640–651. doi:10.2174/1389200211209050640 PMID:22292789

Costache, I. I., Miron, A., Hăncianu, M., Aursulesei, V., Costache, A. D., & Aprotosoaie, A. C. (2019). Pharmacokinetic Interactions between Cardiovascular Medicines and Plant Products. *Cardiovascular Therapeutics*, *9402781*, 1–19. doi:10.1155/2019/9402781 PMID:32089733

Dasgupta, A., Kidd, L., Poindexter, B. J., & Bick, R. J. (2010). Interference of Hawthorn on serum digoxin measurements by immunoassays and pharmacodynamic interaction with digoxin. *Archives of Pathology & Laboratory Medicine*, *134*(8), 1188–1192. doi:10.5858/2009-0404-OA.1 PMID:20670141

David, M. N. V., & Shetty, M. (2021). Digoxin. *StatPearls [Internet]. Treasure Island (FL): StatPearls Publishing.* https://www.ncbi.nlm.nih.gov/books/NBK556025/

Davis, S. A., Feldman, S. R., & Taylor, S. L. (2014). Use of St. John's Wort in potentially dangerous combinations. *Journal of Alternative and Complementary Medicine (New York, N.Y.)*, *20*(7), 578–579. doi:10.1089/acm.2013.0216 PMID:24956073

de Lima Toccafondo Vieira, M., & Huang, S. M. (2012). Botanical-drug interactions: A scientific perspective. *Planta Medica*, *78*(13), 1400–1415. doi:10.1055-0032-1315145 PMID:22864989

Dürr, D. (2000). St John's Wort induces intestinal P-glycoprotein/MDR1 and intestinal and hepatic CYP3A4. *Clinical Pharmacology and Therapeutics*, *68*(6), 598–604. doi:10.1067/mcp.2000.112240 PMID:11180019

Fasinu, P. S., Bouic, P. J., & Rosenkranz, B. (2012). An overview of the evidence and mechanisms of herb-drug interactions. *Frontiers in Pharmacology*, *3*, 69. doi:10.3389/fphar.2012.00069 PMID:22557968

Food and Drug Administration. (2016, December). *Botanical Drug Development: Guidance for Industry*. FDA. https://www.fda.gov/regulatory-information/search-fda-guidance-documents/botanical-drug-development-guidance-industry from https://www.who.int/news-room/factsheets/detail/c ardiovascular-diseases-cvds)

Fugh-Berman, A. (2000). Herb-drug interactions. *Lancet*, *355*(9198), 134–138. doi:10.1016/S0140-6736(99)06457-0 PMID:10675182

Grimstein, M., & Huang, S. M. (2018). A regulatory science viewpoint on botanical-drug interactions. *Yao Wu Shi Pin Fen Xi*, *26*(2), 12–25. doi:10.1016/j.jfda.2018.01.013 PMID:29703380

Izzo, A. A. (2012). Interactions between herbs and conventional drugs: Overview of the clinical data. *Medical Principles and Practice*, *21*(5), 404–428. doi:10.1159/000334488 PMID:22236736

Kim, E. J., Chen, Y., Huang, J. Q., Li, K. M., Razmovski-Naumovski, V., Poon, J., Chan, K., Roufogalis, B. D., McLachlan, A. J., Mo, S. L., Yang, D., Yao, M., Liu, Z., Liu, J., & Li, G. Q. (2013). Evidence-based toxicity evaluation and scheduling of Chinese herbal medicines. *Journal of Ethnopharmacology*, *146*(1), 40–61. doi:10.1016/j.jep.2012.12.027 PMID:23286904

Li, X., Hu, J., Wang, B., Sheng, L., Liu, Z., Yang, S., & Li, Y. (2014). Inhibitory effects of herbal constituents on P-glycoprotein in vitro and in vivo: Herb-drug interactions mediated via P-gp. *Toxicology and Applied Pharmacology*, *275*(2), 163–175. doi:10.1016/j.taap.2013.12.015 PMID:24380838

Lim, X. Y., Chan, J. S. W., Japri, N., Lee, J. C., & Tan, T. Y. C. (2021). Carica papaya L. Leaf: A Systematic Scoping Review on Biological Safety and Herb-Drug Interactions. Evidence-Based Complementary and Alternative Medicine. doi:10.1155/2021/5511221

Lin, H. W., Tsai, H. H., Yu, I. W., Kumar, A., & Wu, M. P. (2014). Would It Matter to Expose Elderly Patients Who Took Digoxin to Chinese Medications? *Value in Health Regional Issues*, *3*, 211–221. doi:10.1016/j.vhri.2014.04.002 PMID:29702930

Liperoti, R., Vetrano, D. L., Bernabei, R., & Onder, G. (2017). Herbal Medications in Cardiovascular Medicine. *Journal of the American College of Cardiology*, *69*(9), 1188–1199. doi:10.1016/j.jacc.2016.11.078 PMID:28254182

Mohammadi, S., Asghari, G., Emami-Naini, A., Mansourian, M., & Badri, S. (2020). Herbal Supplement Use and Herb-drug Interactions among Patients with Kidney Disease. *Journal of Research in Pharmacy Practice*, *9*(2), 61–67. doi:10.4103/jrpp.JRPP_20_30 PMID:33102379

Mueller, S. (2004). Effect of St John's wort dose and preparations on the pharmacokinetics of digoxin*1. *Clinical Pharmacology and Therapeutics*, *75*(6), 546–557. doi:10.1016/j.clpt.2004.01.014 PMID:15179409

Parvez, M. K., & Rishi, V. (2019). Herb-Drug Interactions and Hepatotoxicity. *Current Drug Metabolism*, *20*(4), 275–282. doi:10.2174/1389200220666190325141422 PMID:30914020

Shah, A. U. M., Safri, S. N. A., Thevadas, R., Noordin, N. K., Rahman, A. A., Sekawi, Z., Ideris, A., & Sultan, M. T. H. (2020). COVID-19 outbreak in Malaysia: Actions taken by the Malaysian government. *International Journal of Infectious Diseases*, *97*, 108–116. doi:10.1016/j.ijid.2020.05.093 PMID:32497808

Suroowan, S., & Mahomoodally, F. (2015). Common phyto-remedies used against cardiovascular diseases and their potential to induce adverse events in cardiovascular patients. *Clinical Phytoscience*, *1*(1), 1. doi:10.118640816-015-0002-3

Tachjian, A., Maria, V., & Jahangir, A. (2010). Use of Herbal Products and Potential Interactions in Patients With Cardiovascular Diseases. *Journal of the American College of Cardiology*, *55*(6), 515–525. doi:10.1016/j.jacc.2009.07.074 PMID:20152556

Tankanow, R., Tamer, H. R., Streetman, D. S., Smith, S. G., Welton, J. L., Annesley, T., Aaronson, K. D., & Bleske, B. E. (2003). Interaction Study between Digoxin and a Preparation of Hawthorn (Crataegus oxyacantha). *Journal of Clinical Pharmacology*, *43*(6), 637–642. doi:10.1177/0091270003253417 PMID:12817526

Tsai, H. H., Lin, H. W., Simon Pickard, A., Tsai, H. Y., & Mahady, G. B. (2012). Evaluation of documented drug interactions and contraindications associated with herbs and dietary supplements: A systematic literature review. *International Journal of Clinical Practice*, *66*(11), 1056–1078. doi:10.1111/j.1742-1241.2012.03008.x PMID:23067030

World Health Organization. (2021, June 11). *Cardiovascular diseases (CVDs)*. WHO. https://www.who.int/news-room/fact-sheets/detail/cardio-vascular-diseases-(cvds)

Yu, L. X., Jiang, W., Zhang, X., Lionberger, R., Makhlouf, F., Schuirmann, D. J., Muldowney, L., Chen, M. L., Davit, B., Conner, D., & Woodcock, J. (2015). Novel bioequivalence approach for narrow therapeutic index drugs. *Clinical Pharmacology and Therapeutics*, *97*(3), 286–291. doi:10.1002/cpt.28 PMID:25669762

Chapter 10
What Pharmacological Evidence Exists for Drug-Herbal Interactions on the Human Body?

Joycelyn Chai
Xiamen University Malaysia, Malaysia

Shu Min Chow
Xiamen University Malaysia, Malaysia

Hou Yee Wong
Xiamen University Malaysia, Malaysia

Sock Yan Yap
Xiamen University Malaysia, Malaysia

EXECUTIVE SUMMARY

Chinese herbal medicine is one of the treatment pathways amongst the multicomponent therapeutics of traditional Chinese medicine (TCM). The main role of it includes regaining homeostasis, stabilizing health, preventing illnesses, and overall, prolonging life span and improving quality of life. Since TCM is more focused on treating the root of diseases, Chinese herbal medicine can also be used to prevent, treat, and manage various chronic diseases, such as cardiovascular diseases, musculoskeletal disorders, neurological disorders, and so on. Other significant roles can also be seen as to alleviate several side effects of Western medicine's treatment and be incorporated as part of the management process of the disease recovery and rehabilitation period.

DOI: 10.4018/978-1-6684-7828-8.ch010

INTRODUCTION

Chinese herbal medicine is one of the treatment pathways amongst the multicomponent therapeutics of traditional Chinese medicine (TCM). The main role of it includes regaining homeostasis, stabilizing health, preventing illnesses and in overall, prolonging life span (Dobos & Tao, 2011) and improving quality of life. Since TCM is more focused on treating the root of diseases, Chinese herbal medicine can also be used to prevent, treat, and manage various chronic diseases (Jiang et al., 2011), such as cardiovascular diseases, musculoskeletal disorders, neurological disorders and so on. Other significant roles can also be seen as to alleviate several side effects of Western medicine's treatment and be incorporated as part of the management process of disease recovery and rehabilitation period (Luo et al., 2019).

The definition of drugs can be explained as the substance that brings about a certain or specific change in the body's biologic function through its chemical actions (Katzung, 2018). In the biologic system, drug molecules act as an agonist or an antagonist that binds to a target molecule known as receptor, where it has a regulatory role. In minor cases, drugs can also act as a chemical antagonist that may interact directly with other drugs or herbs. Drugs are usually administered orally or intravenously, where it is concerned with the ADME process, noted as absorption, distribution, metabolism and elimination. Therefore, a useful drug should have the right properties to be utilized as this is a crucial indication of how it is handled appropriately by the body.

Chinese herbal medicine is said to have a better safety profile when compared to pharmaceutical chemicals, however, there are still a few common safety-related concerns (Table 1) due to inappropriate applications of it (Jiang et al., 2011).

Table 1. Safety concerns related to Chinese herbal medicines and its explanation

Common safety related concerns	Explanation
1. Contain toxic compounds	o Identified as heavy metals. o Examples: mercury, copper, lead, cadmium, etc.
2. Contain conventional Western medications	o Usually, undeclared. o Examples: analgesic, antihistamine, diuretics, corticosteroids, antipyretics, etc.
3. Potential adverse effects from herb-drug interactions	o Further deteriorate health and wellbeing. o Due to the lack of comprehensive approach of safety and effectiveness evaluation, and sufficient monitoring.

Herb-drug interactions happen when the effects of drugs are altered due to the presence of another substance (Williamson et al., 2009), like herbal medicines, altering effectiveness or causing adverse effects, leading to therapeutic failure or toxicities. Herb-drug interaction is a double-edged sword and is of concern to both patients and health care practitioners (Table 2).

Table 2. Reasons to assess herb-drug interactions and its explanation

Herb-drug interactions assessment	Explanation
1. Create public awareness and deeper understanding on the issue	o Prevent public from self-diagnosing. o Avoid undocumented adverse herb-drug event.
2. Physicians can further educate themselves	o Adequately diagnose and treat patient. o Prevent hindering of therapy and risk of disease exacerbation.
3. Physicians can provide proper information to patients	o Appropriately dispensing medications. o Guide and advise patients on its interactions.
4. For future development of clinical guidelines	o Develop new therapeutic strategies that combine both TCM and Western herbs. o Produce better health outcomes with minimal side effects.

LITERATURE REVIEW

St. John's Wort & Docetaxel

St John's wort (SJW) is a natural herbal antidepressant, and it was known to treat people with cancer. The constituent of SJW, Hyperforin, activates the pregnane X receptor (PXR), resulting in improved transcription of the transporter ABCB1, also known as P-glycoprotein (P-gp), and CYP3A4. As a result, it induces CYP3A4 and ABCB1, promoting drug substrate metabolism and excretion (Fasinu & Rapp, 2019). Due to CYP3A4 has been discovered that it may be involved in the metabolism of a number of anticancer agents, the bioavailability of intravenous docetaxel, a commonly used anticancer agent for ovarian carcinomas, lung, and breast, was significantly reduced following SJW administration. Docetaxel is a microtubule stabiliser primarily metabolised by CYP3A4 and CYP3A5, resulting in decreased anticancer effectiveness (Geisen & Sturla, 2019). Hyperforin, a SJW ingredient, has been found to accelerate the metabolic and elimination of docetaxel substrates, resulting in reduced of the systemic exposure and thus, also reduces therapeutic efficiency so as the risk of docetaxel-related toxicities (Fasinu & Rapp, 2019).

In ten evaluable cancer patients, the SJW on docetaxel's pharmacokinetics effects were studied (Goey et al., 2013). The pharmacokinetics of docetaxel, which was intravenously administered to all cancer patients on day one of the trials, with 135 mg of docetaxel, were evaluated before and after 14 days with adding 300 mg tablets of

SJW extracts (Hyperiplant) three times daily as supplements. The mean area under the docetaxel concentration-time curve (AUC) of docetaxel was reduced 12% after two weeks of adding the SJW product Hyperiplant as supplements at the advised dosage, indicating decreased systemic exposure of docetaxel. This result was due to the acceleration of the elimination, which has evidence of 14% rise in the clearance of docetaxel after SJW supplementation. The drop in docetaxel AUC observed after SJW supplementation might influence docetaxel's therapeutic effectiveness and toxicities. Hence, administrating SJW to cancer patients on docetaxel might result in undertreatment. Docetaxel's maximum plasma concentration (Cmax) and elimination half-life (T1/2) was also reduced. Remarkably, on the first day of cycle 2, there were two patients who unexpectedly observed a rise in AUC of the docetaxel while simultaneously having the lowest hyperforin levels. Contrastingly, the patients who had the largest drop in AUC of the docetaxel seemed to have the highest levels of hyperforin. The above findings thus provide evidence that hyperforin content in SJW products influences CYP3A4 induction (Goey et al., 2013).

Furthermore, owing to SJW supplementation, this research discovered a decreased risk of docetaxel-related adverse effects, most of which were grade 1 to 2 toxicities. Fatigue, baldness, myalgia, fever and nausea were the most prevalent side effects. These findings supported that SJW mechanical abilities are able to stimulate CYP3A4 and increase substrate metabolism (Goey et al., 2013).

To summarise, the clinical trials above proved that utilising the pharmaceutical SJW product at the suggested dosage reduced systemic docetaxel exposure (Goey et al., 2013). In order to avoid undertreatment of cancer patients who are taking docetaxel, they are strongly not recommended to take SJW products concurrently.

St. John's Wort & Rivaroxaban

The interaction between rivaroxaban and SJW is the second potential drug and Chinese herb that may interact and impact the human body. Rivaroxaban is a factor Xa inhibitor (anticoagulant) that works by selectively, competitively, and reversibly inhibiting clotting factor Xa activity, thereby preventing the blood clots formation (Scholz et al., 2021). The kidney eliminates roughly one-third of the oral rivaroxaban while the rest is metabolised in the liver by CYP3A4, a substrate of P-gp and then excreted in bile or urine (Harder & Graff, 2013).

A single-centre, open-label, and non-randomised was conducted to show the evidence of SJW and rivaroxaban interactions. Twelve healthy adults were enrolled, before each study period (one with and one without preceding CYP induction), CYP3A4 and P-gp phenotyping was done using midazolam and fexofenadine, correspondingly. In healthy individuals, the CYP3A4 and P-gp inducing SJW extract significantly reduced rivaroxaban exposure and pharmacodynamic effect.

The administration of SJW extract containing hyperforin for two weeks reduced the Cmax and exposure (AUC) of rivaroxaban by 14% and 24%, respectively, with a subsequent reduction of a factor Xa inhibition. The geometric mean ratios for rivaroxaban AUC and Cmax pre- and post-induction with SJW extract were 0.76 and 0.86 respectively, indicate a clinically interaction. Factor Xa activity inhibition was decreased with a geometric mean AUC ratio of 0.80 pre- and post-induction. There were no clinically differences in rivaroxaban's Tmax or terminal elimination half-life. Thus, SJW extracts induced the CYP3A4 and P-gp activity significantly (Scholz et al., 2021).

Huppertz et al., also investigate the effect of SJW on the pharmacokinetics of rivaroxaban and macitentan in 2018. Rivaroxaban AUC and Cmax were reduced by 25% when the SJW extract Jarsin® 300 mg was administered three times daily. Macitentan was co-administered with rivaroxaban in conjunction with the SJW extract in this study, rivaroxaban's renal clearance was not affected, proving that the changes were not due to an increase in renal excretion. In the study of Scholaz et al., there is also a similar change in rivaroxaban AUC when macitentan was absent. Scholz et al. study examined possible explanations for the smaller reduction in Cmax, including interindividual variability in rivaroxaban pharmacokinetics, study population differences, or macitentan's effect.

There was no profound adverse effect observed throughout the study. only one transient and mild adverse event occurred, which is the urinary tract infection. Still, it is reported to be unrelated to the medication being used in the trial. From day 4 to day 8 of the clinical trial, subject number 12 was given with ciprofloxacin, that is following phenotyping but concurrent with the first session's rivaroxaban administration (Scholz et al., 2021).

Therefore, the CYP3A4 and P-gp inducing SJW extract caused a significant decrease in rivaroxaban exposure and pharmacodynamic effect of healthy individuals. Despite the absence of contraindication in the combination or systematic adjustment of rivaroxaban administration and dosage, patients taking rivaroxaban in combination with SJW extracts containing hyperforin should be advised not to use the combination or have their plasma concentrations of rivaroxaban monitored (Scholz et al., 2021).

Pomelo & Cyclosporine

Unlike the previous interactions, the following interaction, which is between pomelo and cyclosporine, can improve its medication pharmacokinetics. Pomelo is an expectorant and antitussive in TCM. Pomelo contains furanocoumarins such as dihydroxybergamottin and bergamottin that inhibit CYP3A and P-gp. Allograft rejection and autoimmune illnesses are often treated with cyclosporine, which is a calcineurin inhibitor. Cyclosporine is metabolized by CYP3A and P-gp, so consuming it with pomelo enhances its bioavailability (Anlamlert et al., 2015).

One trial revealed the pharmacokinetics of cyclosporine which, pomelo juice substantially raised cyclosporine concentrations in fourteen young Thai volunteers. Each subject took 2 × 100 mg oral cyclosporine with 200ml water. Then, they were given 250 g pomelo pulp or 250 ml water an hour before and 10 minutes after receiving the medication. Following the administration with pomegranate pulp, it raised cyclosporine's Cmax and AUC by 36.1 and 28.8%, respectively. The higher AUC indicates enhanced systemic exposure to docetaxel, indicating that the active components in pomelo pulp are adequate to enhance the oral bioavailability of cyclosporine (Chen et al., 2018). Compared to the control group, pomelo juice lowered cyclosporine's T1/2.

Minor or transitory adverse effects were reported by 85.7% out of the trial participants, which the flush was the most common adverse effect observed. Fainting and dizziness were also reported. However, it had no severe side effects during the trial (Anlamlert et al., 2015).

To summarise, in healthy participants, pomelo pulp was shown to enhance cyclosporine bioavailability. To reduce the concentration-dependent cyclosporine toxicity, patients who are taking cyclosporine routinely should however avoid consuming pomelo pulp (Anlamlert et al., 2015).

CONCLUSION

In conclusion, depression is perhaps the most prevalent psychiatric disorder in cancer patients. Hence, SJW is helpful to treat mild to moderate depression. However, the use of SJW and docetaxel has elevated the transcription of CYP3A4 and P-glycoprotein. As a result, the metabolism and excretion of drug substrates will increase. Consequently, the systemic exposure to docetaxel is reduced and it led to a decrease in therapeutic efficacy (Goey et al., 2013). Therefore, TCM has emerged as a viable option for cancer patients seeking to improve their quality of life. Jia Wei Xiao Yao San has been found in Taiwan to assist cancer patients in alleviating pathological concerns such as anxiety, dyspepsia, and insomnia, making it a popular prescription formulation for breast and stomach cancer (Cheng et al., 2018).

Another clinical trial also revealed that the use of SJW with rivaroxaban has contributed to a reduction in rivaroxaban exposure followed by a subsequent decrease in the pharmacodynamic efficacy (Scholz et al., 2021). Not only that, but patients also who concomitantly use CYP3A4 inducers (Table 3) with rivaroxaban may decrease the effectiveness of the drug too (Di Minno et al., 2017).

Table 3. A report of herbal supplements that activate CYP3A4

Astragalus mebranaceus	Glycyrrhiza glabra	Isatis indigotica	Poria cocos	Paeonia lactiflo	Ligusticum chuanxion
Rehmannia glutinosa	Ophiopogon japonicas	Atractylodes macrocephala	Lonicera japonica	Fructus gardeniae	Rhizoma ginseng

Previous studies have shown that the consumption of pomelo and cyclosporine results in enhancing cyclosporine bioavailability, which in turn will maximize concentration-dependent cyclosporine toxicity (Anlamlert et al., 2015). Due to the narrow therapeutic window of cyclosporine, Chinese herbs such as grapefruit juice, chamomile, and berberine extracted from *Berberis aristate* or *Coptis chinensi* will increase the plasma concentration of cyclosporine. Therefore, the consumption of either juice or herbs by patients undergoing cyclosporine therapy ought to be cautiously and closely monitored (Colombo et al., 2014).

REFERENCES

Anlamlert, W., Sermsappasuk, P., Yokubol, D., & Jones, S. (2015). Pomelo enhances cyclosporine bioavailability in healthy male Thai volunteers. *Journal of Clinical Pharmacology*, *55*(4), 377–383. doi:10.1002/jcph.430 PMID:25408261

Chen, M., Zhou, S. Y., Fabriaga, E., Zhang, P. H., & Zhou, Q. (2018). Food-drug interactions precipitated by fruit juices other than grapefruit juice: An update review. *Yao Wu Shi Pin Fen Xi*, *26*(2S), S61–S71 . https://doi.org/10.1016/j.jfda.2018.01.009]. .

Chen, T. (2017). Hepatotoxicity of Herbal Supplements Mediated by Modulation of Cytochrome P450. *International Journal of Molecular Sciences*, *18*(11), 2353. https://doi.org/10.3390/ijms18112353

Cheng, Y.-Y., Hsieh, C.-H., & Tsai, T.-H. (2018). Concurrent administration of anticancer chemotherapy drug and herbal medicine on the perspective of pharmacokinetics. *Yao Wu Shi Pin Fen Xi*, *26*(2), S88–S95 . https://doi.org/10.1016/j.jfda.2018.01.003.

Colombo, D., Lunardon, L., & Bellia, G. (2014). Cyclosporine and Herbal Supplement Interactions. *Journal of Toxicology*, *2014*, 145325. https://doi.org/10.1155/2014/145325.

Dobos, G., & Tao, I. (2011). The model of western integrative medicine: The role of Chinese medicine. *Chinese Journal of Integrative Medicine*, *17*(1), 11–20. https://doi.org/10.1007/s11655-011-0601-x. .

Ekor, M. (2014). The growing use of herbal medicines: issues relating to adverse reactions and challenges in monitoring safety. *Frontiers in Pharmacology, 4*. doi:10.3389/fphar.2013.00177

Fasinu, P. S., & Rapp, G. K. (2019). Herbal Interaction with Chemotherapeutic Drugs—A Focus on Clinically Significant Findings. *Frontiers in Oncology, 9*. doi:10.3389/fonc.2019.01356

Geisen, S. M., & Sturla, S. J. (2019). Can Foods or Herbs Alter the Bioavailability of Chemotherapy Drugs? *ACS Pharmacology & Translational Science, 2*(2), 143–146. doi:10.1021/acsptsci.9b00007

Goey, A. K. L., Meijerman, I., Rosing, H., Marchetti, S., Mergui-Roelvink, M., Keessen, M., Burgers, J. A., Beijnen, J. H., & Schellens, J. H. M. (2013). The Effect of St John's Wort on the Pharmacokinetics of Docetaxel. [Retrieved from https://doi.org/10.1007/s40262-013-0102-5]. *Clinical Pharmacokinetics*, *53*(1), 103–110.

Gupta, R. C., Chang, D., Nammi, S., Bensoussan, A., Bilinski, K., & Roufogalis, B. D. (2017). Interactions between antidiabetic drugs and herbs: An overview of mechanisms of action and clinical implications. *Diabetology & Metabolic Syndrome*, *9*(1). https://doi.org/10.1186/s13098-017-0254-9]. .

Harder, S., & Graff, J. (2013). Novel oral anticoagulants: Clinical pharmacology, indications and practical considerations. *European Journal of Clinical Pharmacology*, *69*(9), 1617–1633. https://doi.org/10.1007/s00228-013-1510-z.

Huppertz, A., Werntz, L., Meid, A. D., Foerster, K. I., Burhenne, J., Czock, D., Mikus, G., & Haefeli, W. E. (2018). Rivaroxaban and macitentan can be co-administered without dose adjustment but the combination of rivaroxaban and St John's wort should be avoided. *British Journal of Clinical Pharmacology*, *84*(12), 2903–2913. https://doi.org/10.1111/bcp.13757.

Jiang, M., Zhang, C., Cao, H., Chan, K., & Lu, A. (2011). The Role of Chinese Medicine in the Treatment of Chronic Diseases in China. *Planta Medica*, *77*(09), 873–881. https://doi.org/10.1055/s-0030-1270983.

Kam, P. C. A., & Liew, S. (2002). Traditional Chinese herbal medicine and anaesthesia. *Anaesthesia*, *57*(11), 1083–1089. https://doi.org/10.1046/j.1365-2044.2002.02823.x.

Katzung, B. G. (2018). *Basic & clinical pharmacology* (14th ed.). Mcgraw-Hill Education, Copyright.

Lim, J., Chee, S., Wong, W., He, Q., & Lau, T. (2018). Traditional Chinese medicine: Herb-drug interactions with aspirin. *Singapore Medical Journal*, *59*(5), 230–239. https://doi.org/10.11622/smedj.2018051.

Luo, Y., Wang, C.-Z., Hesse-Fong, J., Lin, J.-G., & Yuan, C.-S. (2019). Application of Chinese Medicine in Acute and Critical Medical Conditions. *The American Journal of Chinese Medicine*, *47*(06), 1223–1235. https://doi.org/10.1142/s0192415x19500629.

Minno, A., Frigerio, B., Spadarella, G., Ravani, A., Sansaro, D., Amato, M., Kitzmiller, J. P., Pepi, M., Tremoli, E., & Baldassarre, D. (2017). Old and new oral anticoagulants: Food, herbal medicines and drug interactions. *Blood Reviews*, *31*(4), 193–203 . https://doi.org/10.1016/j.blre.2017.02.001.

Pasi, A. K. (2013). Herb-Drug Interaction: An Overview. *International Journal of Pharmaceutical Sciences and Research*, *4*(10), 3770–3774. https://doi.org/10.13040/ijpsr.0975-8232.4(10).3770-74.

Scholz, I., Liakoni, E., Hammann, F., Grafinger, K. E., Duthaler, U., Nagler, M., Krähenbühl, S., & Haschke, M. (2021). Effects of Hypericum perforatum (St John's wort) on the pharmacokinetics and pharmacodynamics of rivaroxaban in humans. *British Journal of Clinical Pharmacology*, *87*(3), 1466–1474. https://doi.org/10.1111/bcp.14553.

Singh, A., & Zhao, K. (2017). Herb–Drug Interactions of Commonly Used Chinese Medicinal Herbs. *International Review of Neurobiology*, 197–232. doi:10.1016/bs.irn.2017.02.010

Wachtel-Galor, S. & F., I. (2011). *Herbal Medicine*. Nih.gov; CRC Press/Taylor & Francis. https://www.ncbi.nlm.nih.gov/books/NBK92773/

Williamson, E., Driver, S., & Baxter, K. (2009). *Stockley's herbal medicines interactions: a guide to the interactions of herbal medicines, dietary supplements, and nutraceuticals with conventional medicines*. Pharmaceutical Press.

Chapter 11
A Field Study for Milk Safety and Quality Determination of Heavy Metal Concentration in Raw Milk:
Dairy Science ad Technology

Bardhyl Limani
Faculty of Food Technology and Nutrition, University of Tetovo, North Macedonia

Mohammad Ayaz Ahmad
https://orcid.org/0000-0002-5731-5439
University of Guyana, Guyana

Vesna Karapetkovska Hristova
University of St. Kliment Ohridski, Bitola, North Macedonia

Antalov Jagnandan
University of Guyana, Guyana

Syed Khalid Mustafa
University of Tabuk, Saudi Arabia

Jalal Hasan Baker
University of Tabuk, Saudi Arabia

Samira Jebahi
National Center for Sciences and Nuclear Technologies, BiotechPole, Tunisia

Mohammad Rehan Ajmal
University of Tabuk, Saudi Arabia

Abdul Mosawir Quraishi
Qassim University, Saudi Arabia

EXECUTIVE SUMMARY

In this chapter, a modest attempt has been made to study the heavy metal contamination including their bio-accumulation and toxic effects in our daily lives. It is the alarming hazards to the environment, especially in the industrial zones, that confirm the attention paid to these contaminants. The authors tried to determine the content of

DOI: 10.4018/978-1-6684-7828-8.ch011

heavy metals (cadmium - Cd, lead - Pb, copper - Cu, zinc - Zn, nickel - Ni, manganese – Mn, and chromium - Cr) in the individual samples of cow milk from the farms in seven different localities. The distribution and dynamics of the determined heavy metals in the milk were recorded at different distances starting from the area of the industrial capacity. All the milk samples were analyzed properly, and the authors did chemical consumption and somatic cells and bacteria inside them. The findings were found within good agreements with others.

INTRODUCTION

Nowadays, modern humanity is facing serious environmental challenges and conflicts in its millennial civilization, thanks to unscrupulous actions and deeds. The environmental pollution is a current global problem that poses a serious risk not only to humans but to the entire living world. The rapid pace of urbanization, industrialization and the use of chemicals such as fertilizers, pesticides and drugs, resulting in increased contamination and environmental degradation, leading to a negative effect on the entire living world, disturbing the balance of ecosystems, endangering of human health and other living organisms and intensifying the loss of many vital resources (Mehri, 2004). Further, there are a lot of publications and annual reports, especially by the EU and other developed countries, which clarify that the adverse effects of pollution on humans and animals, in the form of specific chemical toxicity, behavioral changes, or population decline (such as Grue et al., 1997).

The name heavy metals are obtained because their density is higher than 5.0 g / cm^3. The animals and plants absorb from the air, and then through the food has entered the body, where they inhabit the bodies, central nervous system and bones. These compounds are of anthropogenic origin, and their concentration in the environment is increasing due to urban, agricultural and industrial influences. Consequently, controlling the concentration of these elements in food is not only an important indicator of food quality, but also indirectly monitors the impact of these elements on soil, air and water, so that they are the primary indicators of the occurrence of pollution.

Heavy metals do not decompose in the environment, and some are bioaccumulative, i.e., they gradually accumulate in plants and animals and can not be excreted from them. Their non-degradability and potential for long-distance transport into the atmosphere show that the emission of heavy metals into the atmosphere affects even the most remote regions of the source of emissions. (Environmental Quality in RM, 2017 and references therein). Worldwide, more than six billion people use milk and dairy products as a major source of nutrients in the human diet. It is especially important in infant nutrition, as its protein and mineral composition is essential (Buldini et al., 2002). The mineral composition of milk includes several main elements such as calcium, phosphorus and magnesium, as well as potassium, sodium and chlorine and a wide range of trace elements, including zinc, copper, iron, manganese and iodine. Accumulation of heavy metals in the ecosystem (water, soil, plants and animals) causes great toxicity and leads to side effects in living organisms (Bogut et al., 2000). The presence of some polluting metals in the environment, especially cadmium, lead and nickel allows their easy distribution in the food chain, which increases the risk to human and animal health (Licata et al., 2004). Therefore, the presence of high concentrations of heavy metals in dairy products can be a potential risk for serious diseases and public health problems (Pavlovic et al., 2004) and for this reason the determination of heavy metal content in raw milk is an important indicator of the hygienic condition of this product, as well as the level of pollution in the region in which the milk is produced (Licata et al., 2004) & (Ghindini et al., 2005). According to some literature data, cow's milk contains very low concentrations of heavy metals (Lopez et al., 2002), which, however, sometimes increase, although their excretion through milk is proportionally low, but Nwude et al. (2010) found that blood is the major medium for transporting heavy metals in milk, so that milk can certainly be considered as a bio-indicator of industrial pollution.

The selected heavy metals that are the aim of our research: lead (Pb), cadmium (Cd), copper (Cu), zinc (Zn), nickel (Ni), manganese (Mn) and chromium (Cr) are in principle potentially toxic elements if they are present in the food in concentrations that are above the allowed limits and which are also prescribed by the Food and Agriculture Organization (FAO), the World Health Organization (WHO), as well as the legal norms of the Macedonian standards (Official Gazette of RM- No. 102/2013). Data from the literature and numerous studies on the increased presence of heavy metals in milk and dairy products, which often point to a direct link between industrial growth, urbanization and mechanized agriculture, were one of the motivations to begin an extensive research on content determination (Mustafa, 2020; Ayar et al., 2009). of heavy metals in raw milk from farms located in the Polog region, an area where a long-standing industrial pollutant is located.

Unfortunately, additional studies are lacking to allow a detailed examination of the spatial distribution of these contaminants, heavy metals in raw cow's milk.

Therefore, the present study aims to study the distribution of heavy metals at selected milk production sites in the Polog region. This study will contribute to improving the knowledge and information about the current state of this type of milk contamination in the region. This research can be used to clarify the definition of the appropriate sampling procedure for regular control of heavy metal contamination of milk.

Due to the concern about the safety of food of animal origin and thus determining the risk to human health and wildlife that exists in this region and a wider study was conducted at a regional health facility in the Polog Valley on the incidence of respiratory and cancerous diseases in human population and mortality, in the period from 2015-2019.

Through the obtained results, conclusions and recommendations for the public about the state in the Polog region, the environmental awareness of the population will be strengthened as well as the increase of the awareness for consuming safe and quality products such as in our case raw cow's milk.

RESEARCH AIMS AND OBJECTIVES

The problem of heavy metal contamination, their bioaccumulation and toxic effects on wildlife, as one of the alarming hazards of the environment, especially in industrial zones, confirms the attention paid to this type of contaminants. There is also a lack of monitoring and control of heavy metals in water and vegetation, especially in potentially contaminated areas. Numerous studies throughout the world literature determine the content of heavy metals in group tank milk, in terms of nutrition and environmental factors. However, studies on the relationship between milk and feed at the individual level per cow are rare, especially cows raised near sources of contamination.

The main aim of this research is to determine the content of heavy metals (cadmium - Cd, lead - Pb, copper - Cu, zinc - Zn, nickel - Ni, manganese - Mn and chromium - Cr) in individual samples of cow's milk from farms in seven different localities and to determine the distribution and dynamics of the presence of heavy metals in the milk at different distances starting from the industrial area. Additionally, during the research, a total of four (4) alkali metals - macroelements (K-potassium, Ca-calcium, Mg-magnesium, Na-sodium) were analyzed, in samples of milk and fodder.

The determination of these heavy metals in raw milk is of great importance not only for dairies, where the raw material is purchased in terms of its quality and safety, but more for the health of consumers of milk and dairy products, especially the young population - children.

In order to achieve the goals, during the research the following tasks were realized:

1. An observation was made of the eco-climatic conditions specific to the Polog Valley and the pollution that is present in the region.
2. The physico-chemical and microbiological parameters of the examined raw milk samples are determined.

3. The content of heavy metals and alkali metals - macronutrients (K-potassium, Ca-calcium, Mg-magnesium, Na-sodium) in the samples of fodder using atomic absorption spectroscopy was determined and the values were presented, comparing them with the allowed prescribed values by the Law of food safety and products and materials that come in contact with food.
4. The content of heavy metals and macroelements (K-potassium, Ca-calcium, Mg-magnesium, Na-sodium) in the cow's milk samples was determined by atomic absorption spectroscopy, the results were interpreted and the values were compared with those allowed with the effective Law.
5. A survey was conducted on the basis of collecting data from a health institution in the Polog Valley for the condition of respiratory and malignant diseases in the human population for a period of five years (2015-2019), in order to see how environmental pollution and possible presence of heavy metals in milk as a potential factor for the occurrence of diseases in the population that exists in such regions.
6. It is of great importance to raise environmental awareness among the population in the region and throughout the country, as well as awareness and the importance of consuming safe milk with good quality.

MATERIALS AND MEATHODOLOGY

Description of Data Sample Collection

As a working material in this doctoral dissertation is raw cow's milk produced in seven (7) selected farms, dispersed in seven different locations located at an appropriate distance from each other (7-10 km), selected according to the "wind rose" in the Polog region, as which are: Bogovinje (550 m), Janciste (396 m), Jegunovce (396 m), Negotino (575 m), Poroj (500 m) .c), Slatino (540 m) and Toplica (570 m).

According to the geographical location, the farm in Negotino is near the highway Mother Teresa (at a distance of about 30 meters), while the farms from Poroj and Slatino are located near the regional road (about 100-150 meters).

A GIS map of the locations was prepared, from where the samples, altitude, wind rose, relief and infrastructure were taken.

Figure 1. Image of Map used for the collection of Milk Sample from sites

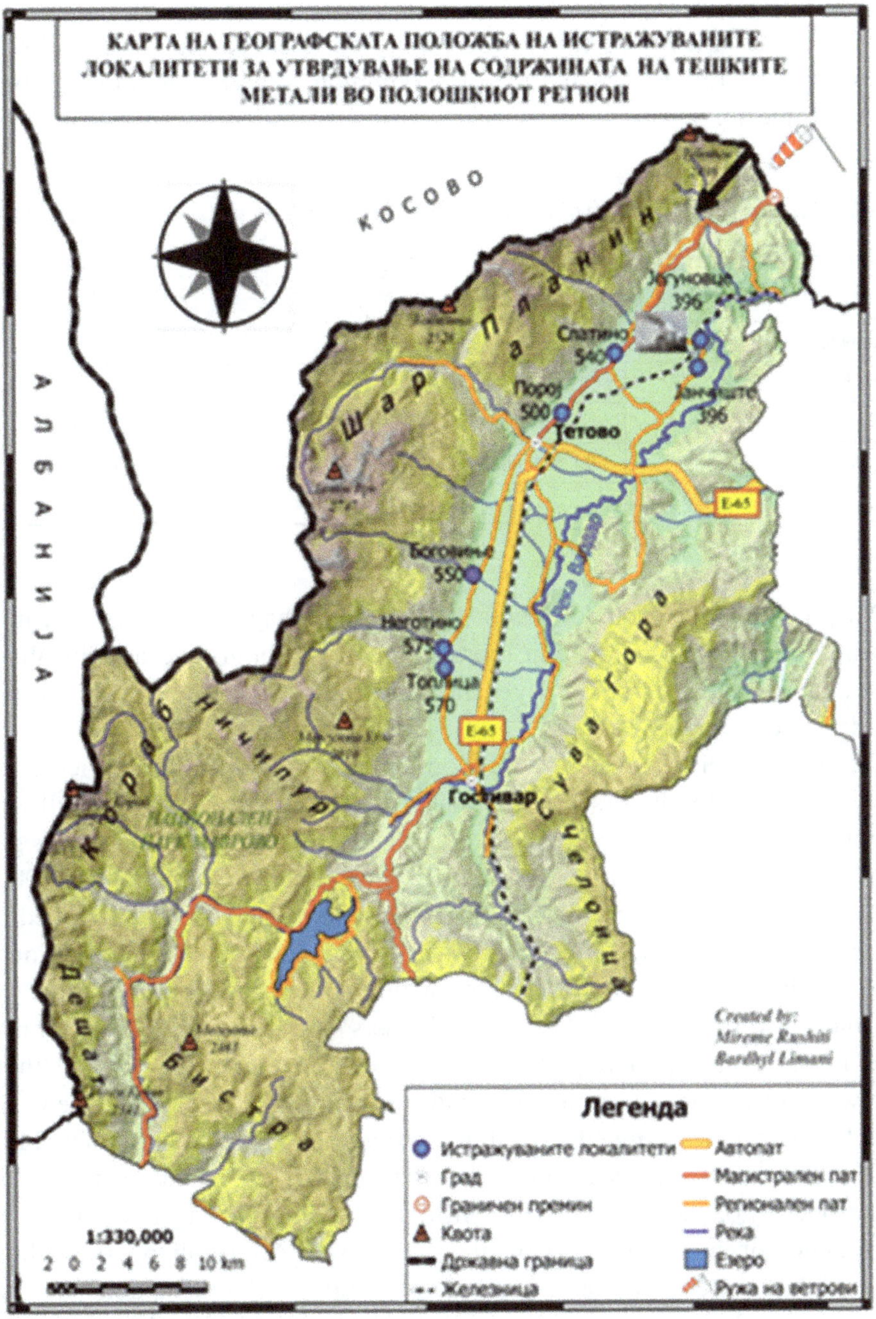

Technology for Dairy Farming

The size of the farms is up to 30 heads, dairy cows are reared in tie -stalls. The cows are of different breeds, but the most common is the Holstein Frisian breed. (See the Table-1).

Table 1. Rations for cows with body weight of 500-600 kg in the farms in Polog region

Livestock feed (kg)	8-12	Milk yield (L) 12-18	18-22	22-27
Meadow hay	2 – 2.2	2.2	2.5	2.6
Alfalfa hay	6-9	8	7.5	8
Corn silage	19	22	22.5-24	24-25
Concentrate (LC)- 18%	5-7 Concentrate - (15%)	10	11- 11.5	12
Straw	1	0.7	0.3	0.3

Dairy cows ration include: alfalfa hay, meadow hay, corn silage and mixed concentrate from own production (corn grain, wheat bran) and additionally the concentrate contains imported soybeans and premixes. The ration for cows has been depicted in Table1.

The diet was distributed in two rations, morning and evening (twice a day), which was manually dispersed in the mangers. The rations consist of bulky feed and concentrate for dairy cows with 16% and 18% protein. The concentrate is given in a mixture with silage during the first and second phase of lactation (0-100 and 100-200 days) and is given only in the evening ration. The farms are supplied with drinking water coming from the rural water supply network system, individually. Water supply is twice a day with buckets or automatic sprinklers. The fodder came from the environment of the farms, the farmers' own production. The food was stored in barns, in a separate part of the barns or stored under canopies. Although the cows in all selected locations were stall-tied keeping system, still in the vicinity of the farms there was limited space for outdoor releasement at least up to 2 hours per day. The calves were separated from the mothers in separate boxes and in a separate facility on the farms. The milking of the cows was mostly mechanical, with the exception of the farms in Bogovinje and Janciste. After milking, the milk was kept in milk lactofreezers (evening and morning milk) until redemption. According to data provided by farmers, the average daily milk yield in all locations ranged from 18-25 liters per head.

Individual milk samples were taken in sterile plastic containers with caps (500 ml) by direct manual milking of the udder, according to a random selection of cows. In addition, 300 ml of milk were separated for physico-chemical composition and microbiological analysis and 200 ml were taken for analysis of heavy metals.

For examination of the physical-chemical and microbiological composition of the milk, five (5) samples were taken from each farm, or a total of 35 samples from the seven (7x5) farms. From the same milk samples, a total of six (6) heavy metals were examined (cadmium - Cd, lead - Pb, copper - Cu, zinc -Zn, nickel - Ni, manganese - Mn) and a total of four (4) alkali metals - macroelements (K-potassium, Ca-calcium, Mg-magnesium, Na-sodium). The samples were taken seasonally, quarterly, which means that a total of 140 milk samples (35 x 4) were analyzed from all farms. Exclusively, the samples for analysis of heavy metals in fodder (individual samples of concentrate and alfalfa hay) from the seven selected farms were performed once during the whole experiment, or a total of seven (7) samples of fodder. The analyzes of the taken feed samples were made by repeating three consecutive tests. The manner of sampling and transport was performed in accordance with the Rulebook on storage of raw milk and sampling for analysis and superanalysis (Official Gazette of the Republic of Macedonia no. 140/10 and 53/11). Also, in the beginning, analyzes were made to determine the concentration of chromium - Cr in milk samples, but the concentration of this element was not detected despite repeated attempts.

PHYSICO-CHEMICAL METHOD FOR DAIRY FARMING

The physico-chemical parameters of milk samples expressed in% (fat, SBM, protein, lactose, minerals, freezing point, density and pH) were tested in the dairy "Eko Shar", Tetovo with Laktoskan apparatus, model Funke Gerber, Type: LactoStar laboratortechnik 12105 Berlin, App- Nr3510-170610. The Funke Gerber Cryostar instrument was used to determine the freezing point of milk and the percentage of water added.

Microbiological Methods

Analysis of Total Number of Somatic Cells and Total Number of Bacteria

Microbiological analyzes of milk (number of somatic cells and total number of microorganisms) were performed in an accredited laboratory for microbiological analysis at the Faculty of Veterinary Sciences in Skopje. Total somatic cell counts were examined with Fossomatic 5000 (Foss Electric, Denmark). The somatic cell counting procedure was performed in accordance with the accredited method ISO 17025- FVM-SOP-398, according to references from ISO 13366-2: 2006. The milk samples were delivered in sterile plastic cups in which the preservative Azidiol (Sigma-Aldrich) in the amount of 0.25 ml was previously added and transported at a temperature of + 4^{0}C to the Laboratory for raw milk quality at the Faculty of Veterinary Medicine - Skopje. It is common practice for samples to be analyzed no later than 72 hours after milk intake. The samples are first heated to a temperature of 40^{0}C for 15 minutes and then analyzed on a Fossomatic 5000 (Foss Electric, Denmark), counting in two repetitions. The microbiological analyzes were performed in an accredited laboratory (comfort standard ISO 17025/2006 from IARM with certificate no. LT-006). Samples for the total number of bacteria were analyzed according to an accredited method, in accordance with ISO-21187: 2004. The Bactoscan 8000 (Foss Electric, Denmark) was used to count the total number of microorganisms, while the procedure was performed according to the Milk-Quantitative determination of bacteriological quality, IDF Standard 161A:1995. The operating principle of this device is staining the bacteria with fluorescent dye. After the bacterial staining procedure, a thin layer (film) of the milk sample, applied to a rotating disk, passes under the lens of a fluorescent microscope. Specifically, this microscope counts colored bacteria as light pulses that are converted electronically and displayed as numerical data.

Determination of the Concentration of Heavy Metals and Macro Elements (Cu, Cd, Pb, Mn, Ni, Zn, K, Mg, Ca, Na)

1. Determination of content of heavy metals and macroelements in milk
2. Determination of content of heavy metals and macroelements in feed

Sampling

After taking the individual samples of raw cow's milk (200 ml / cow) in order to determine the concentration of heavy metals and macronutrients in the milk, they were transported to the Institute of Ecology at the University of Ss. Cyril and Methodius in Skopje. Also, seven (7) samples of fodder were taken for analysis according to the measures of the Rulebook on sampling methods and methods for physical, chemical and microbiological analysis of feed ("Official Gazette of SFRY, no. 15 pp. 423-427, 1987).

Reagents

All reagents were of analytical quality, unless otherwise stated. Milli-Q ultra-pure deionized water type (with a specific resistance of 18.2 $M\Omega cm^{-1}$) was used for all dilutions. HNO_3 and H_2O_2 were of high quality (Sigma-Aldrich). The standard solutions of the elements used for calibration were prepared by diluting a solution of 1000 mg / L of the given element and supplied by the chemical company Sigma-Aldrich.

Apparatus

Agilent Technologies 55 AA Atomic Absorption Spectrometer model with deuterium background corrector was used for the analysis of heavy metals in milk and animal feed. The elements Pb, Cd, and Ni were determined by HGA graphite furnace using high purity argon. The other measurements were performed with a flame air / acetylene technique. The operating conditions and the used program for hitting were carried out according to the instructions recommended by the producer. The elements were extracted from their matrix using nitric acid and hydrogen peroxide in a sand bath.

The preparation of samples and determination of the content of heavy metals in milk and fodder consisted of two laboratory phases:

1) digestion (combustion, decomposition) of the material and
2) determination of the concentration of heavy metals in the digested material by means of atomic absorption spectrometry. The method used for analysis is developed and validated using certified reference material.

Milk was digested using the wet combustion method according to Soylak et al. (2004), covering the following procedures:

- Weighing 5 ml of raw milk into clean and properly labeled flasks for each individual test separately and transfer to Kjeldahl (100 ml) flasks;
- Decomposition / combustion of the material with oxy-acid mixture for organic combustion HNO_3 / H_2O_2 (2: 1) (12 ml for 5 ml sample);
- Setting the flasks in a sand bath and burn them at a temperature of (140°C) for a period of 12 hours, until the contents of the flascks become clear with a light yellow color (maximum 14-16 hours).
- Filtering and transferring combusted material (1-2 ml) in weighing flasks (25 ml) with the addition of distilled water; The blank test was performed in the same way.

- Maintenance of test tubes, with the resulting solutions of combustible material in a refrigerator (4°C), before being used to analyze the content of heavy metals.
- After cooling, the burnt material is diluted with Milli-Q water in a 25 ml glass flask and finally transferred to a previously cleaned and marked polypropylene container for further analysis.
- Each type samples were prepared three digestion and analyzed using three replica.
- Preparation of three blanks.

The same procedure was followed for the preparation of feed samples for analysis.

First, the absorber was calibrated to the 0.2 standard; 0.5 and 2. The concentration of heavy metals in the solutions in the tested tubes was determined using Agilent 55A flame atomic absorption spectroscopy for Cu, Zn and Mn, and Agilent 240 Z graphite atomic absorption spectroscopy for Cd, Pb, Ni and Cr.

The heavy metal content in the samples (γ) was expressed as mg / L and mg / kg or μg / • L and μg / • kg according to the following formula:

$$\gamma = (c \cdot V) - S/m$$

wherein *c* is the concentration of the solution read on the Absorber (ppm or ppb); *V* represents the volume of the combustion solution (25 ml); *S* is the concentration of the element in the blind test (average value of the three blind samples); *m* is the mass of the sample (0.1 - 0.5 g).

Obtained Statistical Results from Soft Computing

Statistically, the results obtained from the conducted studies were interpreted using variation-statistical methods, which are applied for scientific research purposes (ANOVA). The program with which the statistical analyzes are processed is IBM SPSS statistics version 22. The obtained results were processed with the Microsoft EXCEL 2016 package. In order to make a comparison between the obtained data in different seasons, the ANOVA test was used, while the degree of significance was made according to Tukey HSD. The results regarding the presence of heavy metals in milk and feed were processed using the method - descriptive statistics from the program IBM SPSS (V22.0), while the dependence of heavy metals in milk and livestock feed was made using Pearson statistical method correlation.

RESULTS AND DISCUSSIONS

The results of the analyzes for the mean value of the parameters in raw milk according to the standards for assessment of the quality of raw milk are presented in tables and graphs. The obtained results are presented by seasons and by locations from where the samples were taken.

Physico-Chemical Composition of Cow's Milk

In Table 2 are shown the annual mean values from the analyzes made for the physical-chemical composition of the milk from the selected locations (Jegunovce, Janciste, Slatino, Poroj, Bogovinje, Negotino and Toplice).

In different seasons, the mean of the milk fat shows visible differences and the lowest value was registered in winter 3.643%, while the percentage of milk fat was highest in milk produced in summer season 4.809%. The annual mean value of milk fat from all seasons was 4.220%. Mean of non-fat dry matter (NFDM) was the lowest in the milk samples in the winter season 9.036%, while the highest percentage of NFDM was determined in the summer and was 10.540%. The annual mean value of BSM in milk from all seasons was 9.882%. The average value of proteins from different seasons shows small differences and the lowest value was registered in winter 3.418%, while the highest was the percentage of protein in summer milk 3.960%. The annual mean of proteins from all seasons was 3.737%. The average value of lactose was the lowest in milk in the winter months and was 4.688%, and the highest in the examined samples from the summer season was 5.427%. The annual mean value of lactose from all seasons was 5.126%. The mean value of the density of milk from all seasons was 1.031, while the annual average value of the freezing point of milk was - 0.531°C. The mean value for pH of all seasons was 6.750. The mean of the mineral content in the milk samples was the lowest in the winter season 0.662%, while the highest percentage was recorded in the spring season 0.806%. The annual mean of the percentage of minerals in milk was 0.724%.

Regarding the influence of the season on the percentage of milk fat in milk, Vujičić (1985) in his research concluded that it is the lowest in the summer months, and the highest in the beginning of winter and can vary from 0.2 to 0.3%. The experiments were performed on a diet with the same rations throughout the year, and the results showed the same tendency for milk fat to decrease during the summer and increase during the winter.

Table 2. Annual mean value of the parameters for the physico-chemical composition of the milk from the selected locations, by seasons

Parameters (%)	Winter	Spring	Summer	Fall	(x̄)
Fats	3.643	4.420	4.809	4.007	4.220
NFDM	9.036	10.389	10.540	9.563	9.882
Proteins	3.418	3.936	3.960	3.634	3.737
Lactose	4.688	5.416	5.427	4.974	5.126
Density	1.028	1.034	1.033	1.030	1.031
Freezeing point (° C)	-0.444	- 0.597	- 0.575	- 0.510	- 0.531
Minerals	0.662	0.806	0.724	0.704	0.724
pH	6.749	6.740	6.754	6.755	6.750

*NFDM – Non-fat Dry Matter

In our research, the percentage of milk fat is highest in the summer season and lowest in the winter months, which means that our results are opposite to those of the author. Unlike the percentage of milk fat, which is variable and can increase relatively quickly, the percentage of protein increases very slowly (Vujičić, 1985). This is probably due to the fact that protein content is strongly influenced by genotype or breed and changes more slowly under the influence of paragenetic factors. And in our results, for the percentage of protein it can be noticed that the differences between the seasons are 0.5%.

The average values of all parameters of the physico-chemical composition are in the limit values prescribed by the Rulebook (Official Gazette of RM no. 96/11) and are in accordance with the results of other authors (Srbinovska, 2007).

Total Number of Microorganisms And Somatic Cells In Raw Milk From Selected Locations, By Seasons

In the spring season, the highest mean value for the total number of bacteria and somatic cells was registered in the milk samples from Bogovinje (567 x 10^3) and Toplice (436 x 10^3), while the highest value for the total number of somatic cells was determined in Toplice (446 x 10^3) and Bogovinje (368 x 10^3). The lowest values for the total number of bacteria and somatic cells in the spring were determined in Janciste and Slatino (261 x 10^3) while the lowest values for the total number of somatic cells were determined in Jegunovce, Janciste and Slatino (260 x 10^3).

In the summer season, the highest mean value for the total number of bacteria and somatic cells was registered in the samples from Poroj (474 x 10^3), while the highest value for the total number of somatic cells was determined in Negotino (222 x 10^3). The lowest values for the total number of bacteria in summer were determined in Toplice (228 x 10^3) while the lowest values for the total number of somatic cells were determined in Bogovinje (175 x 10^3).

In the autumn season, the highest average value for the total number of bacteria and somatic cells was registered in the milk samples from Bogovinje (577 x 10^3) and Toplice (545 x 10^3), while the highest value for the total number of somatic cells was determined in Slatino (312 x 10^3) and Toplice (295 x 10^3). The lowest values for the total number of bacteria in autumn were determined in Negotino (185 x 10^3), while the lowest values for the total number of somatic cells were determined in Poroj (87 x 10^3).

In Table 3 are shown the annual mean values of the total number of somatic cells and microorganisms in the raw milk samples from the selected locations.

Table 3. Annual mean of the total somatic cell count (TSCC) and total bacteria count (TBC) in raw milk, by locations

Seasons ($\bar{x}$)	Jegunovce (J)		Janciste (Ja)		Slatino (S)		Poroj (P)		Bogovinje (B)		Negotino (N)		Toplice (T)	
	TC SC x 10^3	TCB x 10^3	TC SC x 10^3	TCB x 10^3	TC SC x 10^3	TCB x 10^3	TC SC x 10^3	TCB x 10^3	TC SC x 10^3	TCB x10^3	TC SC x 10^3	TCB x10^3	TC SC x 10^3	TCB x10^3
Spring	260	275	260	261	260	261	275	347	368	567	265	484	446	436
Summer	190	375	194	348	194	348	195	474	175	324	292	411	195	228
Fall	259	340	187	214	312	275	87	192	167	577	155	185	295	545
Winter	330	147	344	157	344	157	330	235	348	290	190	303	285	261

Note: TSCC- total somatic cell count; TBC- total bacteria count

In the winter season, the highest mean value for the total number of bacteria and somatic cells was registered in the milk samples from Negotino (303 x 10^3), while the highest values for the total number of somatic cells were determined in Bogovinje (348 x 10^3). The lowest values for the total number of bacteria in winter were determined in Jegunovce (147 x 10^3) while the lowest values for the total number of somatic cells were determined in Negotino (190 x 10^3).

According to Rulebook 197/2016 and the EU Directive (Council Directive 853/2004EEC), in our research the mean values for the total number of microorganisms did not meet the prescribed criteria. While the mean values for the total number of somatic cells is in accordance with the prescribed criteria up to 400 000 cells / ml.

Figure 1 shows the mean value for the total number of somatic cells and microorganisms in milk samples taken from selected locations in different seasons. The curve for the number of somatic cells is shown in blue, where the highest value is determined in the winter season and is 310 x 10^3 cells / mL, while the lowest value of the number of somatic cells is registered in the summer season and is 205 x 10^3 cells / mL. The values for the total number of microorganisms in the milk on the graph are shown in orange, and it can be seen that the curve decreases from spring (376 x 10^3 CFU / mL) to winter season (221 x 10^3 CFU / mL).

Figure 2. Mean value of the total somatic cell count (TSCC) and total bacteria count (TBC) in raw milk, by seasons

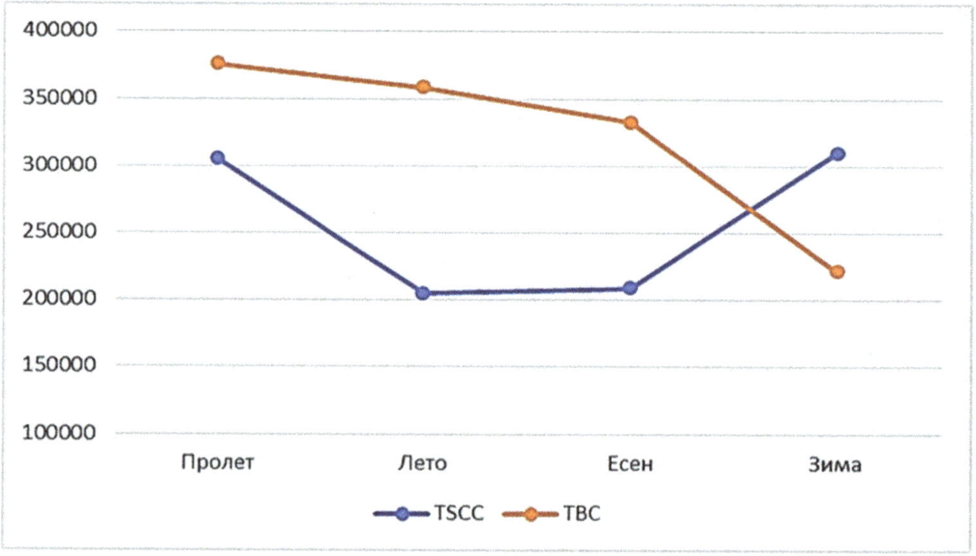

In research conducted by Trajkovska et al. (2016), for the influence of the season on the quality and hygiene of the samples taken from the collective milk from the dairy industry in the Polog region, it was found that the highest value for the total number of somatic cells (TC SC) showed the examined samples in winter season (246.11 x 10^3 cells / mL), while the lowest value was recorded in autumn (237.22 x 10^3 cells / mL). It was also found that the total number of bacteria (TCB) was the lowest in the winter months and was (358.16 x 10^3 CFU / mL), while in the summer season a higher value was registered (365.31 x 10^3 CFU / mL). Our results are in line with those of the authors' research conducted in the same region. In the research of Angelovski and Črceva Nikolovska (2011) the highest mean value for the total number of somatic cells was determined in the summer months. The analyzed samples and the tabulated results clearly indicate insufficient hygiene in the breeding of dairy cows and improper handling of milk after milking as a result of insufficient education of farmers with the hygienic procedures for primary milk production. Contamination of raw milk can come from a variety of sources and types of microorganisms, but it can also be the result of a combination of several factors (unclean equipment and improper cooling of milk). The quality of fresh milk in Kosovo (Bytyqi et al., 2009) still remains quite low compared to existing standards and needs urgent improvement with the application of best practices, advanced and appropriate infrastructure interventions (milking and milk storage equipment, general farm hygiene, storage temperature, etc.).

Content of Heavy Metals and Macronutrients in Raw Cow's Milk by Locations and By Seasons

The results for the content of heavy metals and macroelements of the analyzed milk samples as well as their distribution in the selected locations are presented in Tables 4, 5 and 6. The values are shown through minimum, maximum and average value, as well as the values of standard deviation and standard error.

Table 4. Mean value of the heavy metals and macloelements in raw cow milk from the selected locations by all seasons (Cu, Mn, Zn, K, Ca, Mg, Na - mg/L) and (Cd, Pb, Ni -μg/L)

Heavy Element	J	Ja	S	P	B	N	T
Cu	0096	0.116	0.127	0.141	0.120	0.132	0.160
Cd	0.137	0.106	0.220	0.163	0.425	0.130	0.091
Pb	83.469	26.513	20.713	21.786	32.791	24.865	27.573
Mn	0.115	0.069	0.120	0.143	0.082	0.063	0.092
Ni	34.374	33.985	47.676	36.876	56.167	28.361	31.864
Zn	2.956	2.848	3.399	3.503	3.023	3.416	3.631
K	1306.91	1287.70	1188.387	1171.762	1092.613	1245.675	1315.550
Ca	704.850	152.00	744.645	691.870	964.330	944.525	683.730
Mg	1756.78	2680.100	1979.152	2011.213	1871.917	1863.118	1625.043
Na	343.180	383.016	400.200	363.875	578.295	420.312	348.057

The mean value of copper calculated from all seasons was the lowest in the location Jegunovce and was 0.096 mg / L, while the highest is in Toplice 0.160 mg / L. The cadmium values were lowest in the milk from Toplice 0.091 μg / L / 0.000091 mg / L, and the maximum cadmium concentration was registered in the samples from Bogovinje 0.425 μg / L / 0.000425 mg / L. The mean value of lead showed minimal values in milk from Slatino location 20.713 µg / L / 0.020713 mg / L. The highest lead content was registered in the samples from Jegunovce location 83.469 µg / L / 0.083469 mg / L, as well as in Bogovinje location 32.791 µg / L / 0.032791 mg / L. Taken from all seasons, the mean value of manganese was the lowest in Negotino 0.063 mg / L and in Janciste 0.069 mg / L, while the highest is in Poroj 0.143 mg / L and in Slatino 0.120 mg / L. Maximum values of nickel were registered in the milk from the location Bogovinje 56.167 µg / L / 0.056167 mg / L, and in Slatino 47.676 µg / L / 0.047676 mg / L, and the lowest concentration of nickel was registered in the samples from the location Negotino 28.361 µg / 0.028361 mg / L. The mean values of lead was minimal in the milk samples from Slatino location 20.713 µg / L / 0.020713 mg / L. The highest lead content was registered in the samples from Jegunovce location 83.469 µg / L / 0.083469 mg / L as well as in Bogovinje location 32.791 µg / L / 0.032791 mg / L. The mean value of zinc was lowest in Janciste 2848 mg / L and in Jegunovce 2.848 mg / L, while the maximum content determined in Toplice was 3.631 mg / L and in Poroj 3.503 mg / L. Minimum values of potassium were registered in the milk from the location Bogovinje 1092.613 mg / L, and the highest concentration of potassium was registered in the samples from the location Toplice 1315.550 mg / L and Jegunovce 1306.906 mg / L. The mean value of calcium showed the lowest values in the milk from the location Јанчиштете 152.000 mg / L. The highest calcium content was determined in the samples from the location Bogovinje 964.330 mg / L as well as in the location Negotino 944.525 mg / L.

The values of magnesium were the lowest in the milk from the location Toplice 1625.043 mg / L, and the maximum concentration of this element was registered in the samples from the location Janciste with 2680.101 mg / L. The mean value of sodium showed the lowest values in the samples from Jegunovce 343.180 mg / L and Toplice 348.057 mg / L. The highest sodium content was registered in the milk from the location Bogovinje 578.295 mg / L. Cadmium, lead and mercury are very dangerous to humans and are considered the greatest threat to food in terms of industrial use. In order to determine the content of lead, copper, zinc, mercury and iron in milk samples collected from three different regions, industrial region, rural and high-traffic region around Bursa, Turkey, extensive research was conducted by Simsek et al. (2000). The mean concentrations in the samples from these three regions were as follows: for lead 0.032, 0.049, 0.018 mg / kg; for zinc 4.49, 5.01, 3.77 mg / kg; for copper 0.58, 0.96, 0.39 mg / kg; and for Fe 1.78, 4.27, 1.01 mg / kg, while no mercury was detected in the samples. The highest content of heavy metals is found in milk samples collected from the industrial region, followed by heavy traffic and also in the rural region. The aim of the research of Vlasaku et al. (2017) was to assess the possible contamination of heavy metals in milk from different farms, in three cities (Kumanovo, Tetovo, Gostivar) in Macedonia. Quantitative analyzes of Cd, Cr, Cu and Pb performed using a graphite furnace atomic absorption spectrophotometer showed that the concentration of selected metals was low (<0.1 mg / kg) such as: As, Co, Cd, Cr, Cu, Fe, Pb and Zn. Our results are similar to the results published by the authors, with the exception of the lead content which in the milk samples is above the permitted prescribed values.

In a study by Abolfazl et al. (2012) using atomic absorption spectrometry (AA 220) examined the presence of Pb and Cd in a total of one hundred (100) milk samples taken from different locations in East Azerbaijan: Tabriz, Sarab, Marage, Mejane, Azarshar, Osko, Malekan and Ahar. According to this study, the amount and level of Pb and Cd in cow's milk samples is as follows: the highest cadmium concentration was found in Sarab (4.52 µg / L) and the lowest in the Malekan region (0.57 µg / L / 0.00057 mg / L). The highest concentration of lead was registered in the city of Meyane (182.08 µg / L / 0.18208 mg / L) and the lowest in Ahar (12.82 µg / L / 0.01282 mg / L). Statistical analyzes have shown that there are significant differences between the concentrations of lead and cadmium in raw cow milk samples from different regions of East Azerbaijan. In all samples, the measured cadmium content was less than the permissible limit according to the FAO / WHO authorized limits (Cd: 10 µg / kg / 0.01 mg / kg). However, only in 28% of the samples the measured lead content was lower than the prescribed limit according to the FAO / WHO standard (Pb: 20 µg / kg = 0.02 mg / kg). The presence of heavy metals in milk and dairy products is considered to be due to industrialization as one of the most important contaminants. In our research, the highest cadmium content was registered in Bogovinje 0.425 µg / L / 0.000425 mg / L, and the lowest value in the samples from Toplice 0.091 µg / L / 0.000091 mg / L, but the values do not exceed the prescribed permissible limits according to FAO / WHO. The lead content was above the permissible limits, with the highest value being 83.469 µg / L / 0.08469 mg / L, in the location Jegunovce, while the lowest concentration was determined in the location Slatino and was 20.713 µg / L / 0.020713 mg / L. In the study of Pavlovic et al. (2004)[7], the Pb level ranged from 0.028 to 0.036 µg / mL, while the Cd level was between 0.005 and 0.006 µg / mL for more than 15 farms in Croatia. Sikrić et al. (2003) reported an even higher concentration of Pb in milk, ranging from 0.023 to 0.070 µg / mL.

Lead levels in 1. 20% of the collected samples (12 samples from 997) were above the maximum residual limit imposed by the European Union (0.02 mg / kg) (EC, 2015). In our results for the annual mean of the selected elements we found that the content of all elements except lead was within the normal prescribed permissible limits.

The distribution of lead in milk was in the following order of locations: J> B> T> Ja> N> P> S. Mean lead levels from all seasons ranged from 0.021 to 0.083 mg / L, from where the maximum mean values were determined in Jegunovce and

Bogovinje. As for the cadmium content in the milk samples, it was below the allowed prescribed values and had the following distribution by locations, as follows: B> S> P> J> N> Ja> T. For the copper content from Table 5, the following distribution of this element by locations can be concluded as follows: T> P> N> S> B> Ja> J. The distribution of manganese by locations was in the following order P> S> J> T> B> Ja> N. From all seasons the distribution of manganese by locations followed the order: P> J> T> B> Ja> N. The concentration of nickel in the milk samples from the selected locations was determined in the following order: B> S> P> J> Ja> T> N. The distribution of zinc in the analyzed samples had a decreasing content as follows: T> P> N> S> B> J> Ja. The elements such as potassium, calcium, magnesium and sodium in milk had the following order of locations: (K) - T> J> Ja> N> S> P> B; (Ca) - B> N> S> J> P> T> Ja; (Mg) - Ja> P> S> B> N> J> T; (Na) - B> N> S> Ja> P> T> J. Regarding the content of macroelements, they largely depend on the composition of the concentrates, the way of storage and preservation of bulky feeds, as well as the additives in the feed mixtures (premixes and vitamin-mineral supplements). In a study by Zhou Xuewei (2019) found that the mean levels of Pb in milk produced in the ten studied areas show a declining content as follows: E> D> A> G> J> C> B> F> H> I Mean Cd levels ranged from 0.02 to 0.09 μg / L, (0.00002 - 0.00009 mg / L) and the highest mean content was found in areas J and A. Maximum Pb levels were recorded in a sample of area C, while Cd was highest in area J.

Table 5. Sequence of locations according to the concentration of heavy metals and macroelements (from highest to lowest mean value) in raw cow's milk for selected locations of all seasons (Cu, Mn, Zn, K, Ca, Mg, Na - mg / L) and (Cd, Pb, Ni -µg / L)

	T	P	N	S	B	Ja	J
Cu	0.16	0.141	0.132	0.127	0.12	0.116	0.096
	B	**S**	**P**	**J**	**N**	**Ja**	**T**
Cd	0.425	0.22	0.163	0.137	0.13	0.106	0.091
	J	**B**	**T**	**Ja**	**N**	**P**	**S**
Pb	83.469	32.791	27.573	26.513	24.865	21.786	20.713
	P	**S**	**J**	**T**	**B**	**Ja**	**N**
Mn	0.143	0.12	0.115	0.092	0.082	0.069	0.063
	B	**S**	**P**	**J**	**Ja**	**T**	**N**
Ni	56.167	47.676	36.876	34.374	33.985	31.864	28.361
	T	**P**	**N**	**S**	**B**	**J**	**Ja**
Zn	3.631	3.503	3.416	3.399	3.023	2.956	2.848
	T	**J**	**Ja**	**N**	**S**	**P**	**B**
K	1315.55	1306.906	1287.7	1245.675	1188.387	1171.762	1092.613
	B	**N**	**S**	**J**	**P**	**T**	**Ja**
Ca	964.33	944.525	744.645	704,85	691.87	683.73	152.0
	Ja	**P**	**S**	**B**	**N**	**J**	**T**
Mg	2680.10	2011.213	1979.152	1871.917	1863.118	1756.776	1625.043
	B	**N**	**S**	**Ja**	**P**	**T**	**J**
Na	578.295	420.312	400.2	383.016	363.875	348.057	343.18

Annual Mean Value of Heavy Metals and Macro Elements According to The Obtained Results by Seasons from All Locations

The annual mean value of heavy metals and macroelements according to the results obtained by seasons from all locations, and the curve of their distribution are shown in Table 6.

From the Table 6, it has been found that the lowest average value of copper obtained during the analysis of milk samples from all seven locations, by seasons, was determined in the winter season and was 0.093 mg / L, while the highest average value was registered in the summer season 0.151 mg / L. The calculated annual mean value of copper from all seasons is 0.128 mg / L. During the analysis of milk samples from the selected locations by seasons, the lowest mean value for cadmium was determined in the spring season and was 0.078 µg / L / 0.000078 mg / L, while the highest mean value was registered in the winter season 0.351 μg / L / 0.000351 mg / L. The annual mean value of cadmium calculated from all seasons was 0.183 μg / L / 0.000183 mg / L. From the data in the table, for lead the lowest mean value of the seasons was registered in the spring season 9.418 μg / L / 0.009418 mg / L, while the highest value was determined in the winter season and was 61.854 μg / L / 0.061854 mg / L. The calculated annual mean value of lead from all seasons is 35.937 μg / L /0.035937 mg / L. The lowest mean value of manganese obtained during the analysis of milk samples by seasons was determined in the fall season and was 0.036 mg / L, while the highest mean value was determined in the winter season 0.156 mg / L. The annual mean value of manganese from all seasons was 0.098 mg / L. According to the results obtained from the analysis of milk from the selected locations by seasons, the lowest mean value for nickel was determined in the spring season and was 72.350 μg / L / 0.07235 mg / L, while the highest mean value was registered in the fall season 10.776 μg / L / 0.010776 mg / L. The annual mean value of nickel calculated from all seasons was 39.173 μg / L / 0.039173 mg / L. For zinc content, the lowest mean value of milk samples by seasons was determined in spring and was 2.953 mg / L, while the highest mean value was registered in fall season 3.604 mg / L. Otherwise, the annual mean of zinc from all seasons together was 3.283 mg / L. The lowest mean value for zinc content of milk samples by seasons was determined in spring and was 2.953 mg / L, while the highest average value was registered in fall season 3.604 mg / L. Otherwise, the annual mean of zinc from all seasons was 3.283 mg / L.

Górska et al. (2007) found that the concentration of lead in cow's milk was 0.003 mg / kg. In other European countries, the Pb content in milk (mg / kg) was as follows: Slovenia - 0.05 and Spain - 0.0018 (Cerkvenik et al., 2000), Austria - 0.0065 (Pilsbacher & Grubhofer, 2002), Italy - 0.0013 (Licata P., 2004)[6] and Romania - from 0.052 to 0.617 mg / kg (Boltea et al., 2008). In previous studies by Limani et al. (2019) in the Polog region, the average value of lead in the period January - May was 278.21 μg / L / 0.27821 mg / L. Otherwise, in research done by Anastasio et al. (2006) also reported increased levels of cadmium and lead in samples of milk originating in Italy.

Table 6. Annual mean value of heavy metals and macroelements according to the obtained values by seasons from the locations (Cu, Mn, Zn, K, Ca, Mg, Na - mg / L) and (Cd, Pb, Ni -µg / L)

	Winter	Spring	Summer	Fall	x̄
Cu	0.093	0.137	0.151	0.132	**0.128**
Cd	0.351	0.078	0.125	0.176	**0.183**
Pb	61.854	9.418	28.689	43.787	**35.937**
Mn	0.156	0.072	0.129	0.036	**0.098**
Ni	33.429	72.350	40.138	10.776	**39.173**
Zn	3.347	2.953	3.229	3.604	**3.283**
K	1125.000	1226.071	1157.817	1398.629	**1226.879**
Ca	2675.586	114.779	270.563	111.443	**793.093**
Mg	165.000	2140.520	2417.845	2814.571	**1884.484**
Na	361.286	473.814	378.023	391.293	**401.104**

Comparison Between Seasons for The Content of Heavy Metals and Macronutrients in Milk Samples from All Locations (Anova test)

The soft computing by ANOVA statistics simulation was done and was found within the satisfactory of significance at the level 0.05. The differences between the mean values of elements in different seasons have been described such as:

There is no significant difference in the copper content of milk between the mean values in different seasons. For the presence of cadmium in milk, significant differences were found in the mean values at the level of 0.05. The differences between the mean values are significant in the seasons spring - winter (0.27114 *) and summer - winter (0.22629 *).

For lead content in milk is determined significant differences in the mean level of 0.05. The differences are significant in the seasons spring-winter (52.86771 *), summer-winter (33.16571 *) and fall-spring (34.80029 *).

The differences between the mean values of manganese in milk show a significance level of 0.05. There are significant differences between the seasons spring - winter (34.56429 *), autumn - winter (22.65229 *), summer - spring (27.85514 *), fall - spring (57. 21657 *), fall - summer (29.36143 *).

For nickel content in milk is determined significant differences in the mean level of 0.05. The differences are significant in the seasons spring-winter (34.56429 *), fall -winter (22.65229 *), summer-spring (27.85514 *), fall-spring (55.21657 *) and fall -summer (29.36143 *).

For the presence of zinc in milk, significant differences were found in the mean values at the level of 0.05. The differences between the mean values are significant in the spring-fall season (0.65057 *).

In terms of potassium content in milk, the differences between the mean values are significant in the seasons fall -winter (273.62857 *), fall -spring (172.55714 *) and fall -summer (240.81143 *).

Significant differences in mean values of calcium in milk were found at the level of 0.05. The differences between the mean values are significant in the seasons spring-winter (2560.80714 *) and summer-winter (2405.02286 *) fall-winter (2564.14286 *).

Also, for the concentrations of magnesium in milk, significant differences were found between the mean values in the seasons spring-winter (1975.52000 *) and summer-winter (2252.84514 *) fall -winter (2649.57143 *), summer-spring (277.32514 *) and fall - spring (674.05143 *).

For the sodium content in milk, significant differences were found in the mean values at the level of 0.05. The differences are significant in the spring-winter seasons (112.52857*).

In terms of cadmium, one of the most important ways of introducing significant amounts of this metal is through inhalation of contaminated air. In the case of milk, an important source of cadmium is animal feed or manure. The concentration of cadmium in milk is expected to increase with increasing age of the animals (Mahmoudi et al., 2017). However, some studies show that the concentrations of cadmium in cow's milk, which are grazed in industrial areas along highways or in animals fed on heavy metal contaminated feed, are much higher than those grown in ecological areas (Mahmoudi., Et al.2017).

In a study by Tizhoosh M., &. Tizhoosh H. R., (2016) examined the concentration of heavy metals, including zinc, lead, cadmium, and copper in raw milk produced by the dairy industry in Koramabad, Iran. The results showed that the mean concentrations (mg / L) were 3.07 (Zn), 2.72 (Pb), 0.1 (Cd) and 0.14 (Cu). The results of the comparison of the mean concentrations measured with WHO guidelines showed statistically significant difference ($p < 0.05$) suggesting that the average concentration of each element in the studied sample is greater than the WHO recommendations, mainly due to the release of heavy metals through feed and drinking water. In conclusion, the authors conclude that it is necessary to regulate the quality and safety of feed to prevent the release of heavy metals in the dairy and obviously in the human food chain.

HEAVY METAL CONTENT IN FEED

The outcomes for the content of heavy metals and macronutrients in the feed obtained from three consecutive measurements from each location individually have been depicted in Table7. The table also gives the average value of all elements from all locations.

Table 7. Mean value of heavy metals and macronutrients in the feed for the selected locations (Cu, Mn, Zn, K, Ca, Mg, Na - mg / kg) and (Cd, Pb, Ni -µg / kg)

	J	Ja	S	P	B	N	T	x̄
Cu	1.694	1.639	3.171	1.742	3.147	2.119	17.010	**4.360**
Cd	2.417	0.968	7.556	1.667	11.966	3.465	11.498	**5.648**
Pb	29.405	33.290	58.220	19.412	15.239	18.950	63.603	**34.017**
Mn	4.037	5.664	25.220	4.678	17.537	4.214	98.298	**22.807**
Ni	34.308	40.453	62.157	198.637	84.679	73.539	23.357	**73.876**
Zn	19.562	22.408	25.790	19.138	23.133	16.157	100.693	**32.412**
K	2700.00	3080.00	4110.000	2730.00	3750.00	2830.00	4480.00	**3382.857**
Ca	8960.00	9280.00	13940.00	14400.00	8210.00	7050.00	12610.00	**10635.71**
Mg	960.00	1070.00	1230.00	1120.00	1200.00	830.00	2380.00	**1255.714**
Na	110.00	80.000	820.000	400.000	1450.00	70.000	1680.000	**658.571**

Regarding the content of copper (Cu) in the feed, the lowest value was registered in Janciste 1.639 mg / kg, while the highest value was determined in Toplice 17.010 mg / kg. As for the mean of copper calculated from all locations is 4.360 mg / kg. The cadmium content is at least present in the samples of fodder from Janciste 0.968 µg / kg / 0.000968 mg / kg. The highest concentration of this heavy metal was registered in the samples from Bogovinje 11.966 µg / kg / 0.011966 mg / kg and Toplice 11.498 µg / kg / 0.011498 mg / kg. The mean value of cadmium in feed from all locations was 5.648 µg / kg / 0.005648 mg / kg. The content of lead in the fodder is the lowest in Bogovinje 15.239 µg / kg / 0.015239 mg / kg, while the highest value is registered in Toplice 63.603 µg / kg / 0.063603 mg / kg. The mean value for lead calculated from all locations is 34.017 µg / kg / 0.034017 mg / kg. The highest value for manganese is registered in Toplice 98.298 mg / kg, while the lowest in Jegunovce 4.037 mg / kg. The mean value of manganese from all locations is 22.807 mg / kg. The lowest nickel content was determined in Toplice 23.357 µg / kg / 0.023357 mg / kg, and the highest value was registered in Poroj 198.637 µg

/ kg / 0.198637 mg / kg. The mean value of nickel from all locations is 73.876 µg / kg / 0.073876 mg / kg. Zinc in animal feed is least present in the samples from Negotino 16,157 mg / kg, while it is most present in the feed from Toplice 100.693 mg / kg. As for the mean value of zinc from all locations, it is 32.412 mg / kg.

The lowest content of potassium in the feed was determined in Jegunovce 2700.00 mg / kg, and the highest value shows 4480.00 mg / kg, in the samples of fodder taken from the location Toplice. The mean of potassium from all locations is 3382.857 mg / kg. Calcium shows the lowest value in the feed from Toplice 7050.00 mg / kg, and the highest content is present in the samples from Poroj 14400.00 mg / kg. Otherwise, the mean of calcium in animal feed from all selected locations is 10635.710 mg / kg. The highest content of magnesium in the taken feed samples is in Toplice 2380.00 mg / kg and the lowest in the feed samples from Negotino 830.00 mg / kg.

The mean value of sodium in the feed samples from all selected locations was 658.571 mg / kg. Sodium shows the lowest value in the feed from Negotino 70.00 mg / kg, and the highest content is present in the samples from Toplice 1680.00 mg / kg.

Vllasaku (2017) examined the content of some chemical elements (arsenic, cadmium, cobalt, chromium, copper, iron, manganese, nickel, lead, vanadium and zinc) in the feed (concentrate for animal feed and alfalfa and straw silage) from the regions of Kumanovo, Tetovo and Gostivar in the Republic of Macedonia.

The content of heavy metal elements As, Cd, Co, Cr, Ni and Pb was found to be less than 1 mg / kg in all analyzed samples. It was determined that the content of other elements (Cu, Fe, Mn, V and Zn) is lower in the samples for the feed from Kumanovo region than in those from the Tetovo and Gostivar region. Bilandzic et al. (2011) studied the Pb concentration in raw cow's milk in the southern and northern regions of Croatia and found 58.7 µg / L and 36.2 µg / L, respectively. They noticed that the Pb content in the samples taken from both regions exceeded the highest recommended level. In another study, it was found that the Pb content values in milk samples tested in Yugoslavia ranged between 0.00 and 0.02 mg / kg. In a study conducted in an urban area, Yoon et al. (2006) investigated the transfer of lead from automobiles to feed and reported that the concentration of Pb in dry matter was above the maximum limits. If under normal conditions the milk has no contact with the lead material during production and processing, lead contamination does not occur. Lead is a pollutant that comes mostly from the environment and exists in almost all industrial environments.

Correlation Between the Content of Heavy Metals in Feed and Raw Milk

From Table 9 it can be seen that there is a very weak positive correlation (r = 0.125) between fodder copper and milk. There is no statistical significance between the values of copper in feed and milk. It can also be found that there is a weak positive correlation between cadmium in feed and milk (r = 0.169). The correlation is significant at the level of 0.05 (two-way correlation). Regarding the correlation with the element lead, it can be determined that there is a very weak negative correlation between lead in animal feed and milk (r = - 0.062). There is no statistical significance between the values of lead in animal feed and milk. Between manganese in the feed and milk has a very weak negative correlation (r = - 0.017), and while there is no statistical significance. Also from the above table it can be determined that there is a very weak positive correlation between the nickel content in the feed and milk (r = 0.008). There is no statistical significance between the given values. Regarding the element zinc, it can be determined that there is a weak positive correlation between zinc in feed and milk (r = 0.1694). There is no statistical significance among the given values. From the statistical analysis of the macroelements it can be determined that there is a very weak negative correlation between potassium, calcium and magnesium in feed and milk (r = - 0.017; -0.075; -0.084). There is no statistical significance between the values of the selected items in animal feed and milk. From the obtained results it can be determined that there is a weak positive correlation between sodium in feed and milk (r = 0.169). The correlation is significant at the level of 0.05. In a study examining toxic heavy metals in milk and fodder from urban and rural areas by Bushra Iftikhar et al. (2014) found that the concentrations of cadmium, copper, lead, and nickel in milk were higher than the maximum permissible residue limits prescribed by FAO and WHO, while in the feed samples they were within the normal range, meaning that milk was contaminated from other sources but not from the feed. In our research there is a very weak negative correlation between lead in feed and milk (r = - 0.062).

In our research, the content of cadmium, copper, and nickel in cow's milk, although below the limits allowed by the WHO, still found a difference between the values for these elements in the selected locations. Increased levels of these elements were registered in the milk from the farms located in the locations that are more developed in rural areas and which are close to the highway and the regional road, the highest in Bogovinje, Poroj and Slatino, respectively. Regarding the lead content, increased concentrations were registered in relation to the prescribed permissible concentrations and the highest were registered in Jegunovce (0.083469 mg / L), Bogovinje (0.032791 mg / L) and Toplice (0.026513 mg / L).

CONCLUSION

1. Regarding the results of physico-chemical composition of raw cow's milk obtained from the analyzed samples from the selected locations for all seasons, it can be concluded that the mean annual values from the selected locations of all parameters of the physico-chemical composition of raw cow's milk were in the limit values prescribed by the Rulebook.
    - The annual mean of milk fat from all seven locations shows visible differences and the lowest value is determined in Toplice 2.4305%, while the highest percentage of milk fat in the samples of milk produced in the farm in Jegunovce 5.5025%.
    - The percentage of non - fat dry matter (NFDM) is the lowest in the milk samples from Bogovinje and Toplice 8.8725 and 8.9035%, while the highest percentage of NFDM is determined in the milk from Jegunovce and Poroj 10.771 and 10.4035%.
    - The mean value of proteins from all seasons is the lowest in Bogovinje 3.335%, while the highest value from all locations is determined in the milk samples from Jegunovce 4.050%.
    - The annual mean value of lactose is the lowest in the milk from Bogovinje 4.618%, and the highest in the examined samples from Jegunovce 5.5465%.
    - The mean value of milk density ranges from 1.02922 to 1.033405 while the freezing point of milk is in the range of - 0.4073 to - 0.57685 00C. The average pH ranges from 6.7235 to 6.788.
    - The annual mean value of the presence of minerals in the milk samples is the lowest in Jegunovce 0.6825%, while the highest is in the milk from Toplice 0.752%.2.
    - The values for the total number of microorganisms did not meet the prescribed criteria according to According to Rulebook 197/2016 and the EU Directive (Council Directive 853/2004 EEC). While the mean values for the total number of somatic cells is in accordance with the prescribed criteria up to 400 000 cells / ml.
2. According to the results on the influence of the season on the total number of somatic cells and microorganisms, it can be concluded that the season has an impact on the parameters for hygienic quality of the raw milk. The highest value for somatic cells is determined in the winter season and is 310 x 10^3 cells / mL, while the lowest value of the number of somatic cells is registered in the summer season and is 205 x 10^3 cells / mL. The values for the total number of microorganisms in the milk are the highest in the spring season (376 x 10^3

CFU / mL) and the values are the lowest in the winter season (221 x 10^3 CFU / mL).

3. According to the obtained results for the mean values of heavy metals and macroelements in raw milk for the selected locations from all seasons, we concluded the following:
    - The mean of copper calculated from all seasons was the lowest in the location Jegunovce and is 0.096 mg / L, while the highest is in Toplice 0.160 mg / L. Mean values of cadmium were lowest in the milk from Toplice 0.091 μg / L / 0.000091 mg / L, and maximum cadmium concentration was registered in the samples from Bogovinje 0.425 μg / L / 0.000425 mg / L.
    - Mean values of cadmium were lowest in milk from Toplice 0.091 μg / L / 0.000091 mg / L, and maximum cadmium concentration was registered in the samples from Bogovinje 0.425 μg / L / 0.000425 mg / L.
    - Of all seasons, the mean value of manganese was the lowest in Negotino 0.063 mg / L and in Janciste 0.069 mg / L, while the highest is in Poroj 0.143 mg / L and in Slatino 0.120 mg / L.
    - Maximum values of nickel were registered in the milk from the location Bogovinje 56,167 μg / L / 0.056167 mg / L, and in Slatino 47,676 μg / L / 0.047676 mg / L, and the lowest concentration of nickel was registered in the samples from the location Negotino 28,361 μg / 0.028361 mg / L).
    - Regarding the mean of zinc, it was lowest in the location Janciste 2848 mg / L and in Jegunovce 2,848 mg / L, while the maximum content determined in Toplice was 3,631 mg / L and in Poroj 3,503 mg / L.
    - Minimum values of potassium were registered in the milk from the location Bogovinje 1092.613 mg / L, and the highest concentration of potassium was registered in the samples from the location Toplice 1315.550 mg / L and Jegunovce 1306.906 mg / L.
    - The mean value of calcium showed the lowest values in the milk from the location Janciste 152.00 mg / L. The highest calcium content was determined in the samples from the location Bogovinje 964.330 mg / L as well as in the location Negotino 944.525 mg / L.
    - The values of magnesium were the lowest in the milk from the location Toplice 1625.043 mg / L, and the maximum concentration of this element was registered in the samples from the location Janciste 2680.101 mg / L.
    - The mean value of sodium showed the lowest values in the samples from Jegunovce 343.180 mg / L and Toplice 348.057 mg / L. The

highest sodium content was registered in the milk from the location Bogovinje 578.295 mg / L.

4. According to Anova statistics for examining the differences between the mean values of the elements in different seasons:
    - There is no significant difference in the copper content of milk between the mean values in different seasons. For cadmium in milk, significant differences were found in the mean values at the level of 0.05. The differences between the mean values are significant in the seasons spring - winter (0.27114*) and summer - winter (0.22629*).
    - For lead content in milk samples is determined significant differences in the mean level of 0.05. The differences are significant in the seasons spring-winter (52.86771*), summer-winter (33.16571*) and fall-spring (34.80029*).
    - The differences between the mean values of manganese in milk show a significance level of 0.05. There are significant differences between the seasons spring - winter (34.56429*), fall - winter (22.65229*), summer - spring (27.85514*), fall - spring (57. 21657 *), fall - summer (29.36143*).
    - For the nickel content in milk, significant differences were found in the mean values at the level of 0.05. The differences are significant in the seasons spring-winter (34.56429*), fall-winter (22.65229*), summer-spring (27.85514*), fall-spring (55.21657 *) and fall-summer (29.36143*).
    - For the zinc content in milk samples, significant differences were found in the mean values at the level of 0.05. The differences between the mean values are significant in the spring-fall seasons (0.65057 *).
    - In terms of potassium content in milk, the differences between the mean values are significant in the seasons fall-winter (273.62857*), fall-spring (172.55714*) and fall-summer (240.81143*).
    - Significant differences in mean values of calcium in milk were found at the level of 0.05. The differences between the mean values are significant in the seasons spring-winter (2560.80714*) and summer-winter (2405.02286*) fall-winter (2564.14286*).
    - Also, for the concentrations of magnesium in milk, significant differences were found between the mean values in the seasons spring-winter (1975.52000*) and summer-winter (2252.84514*) fall-winter (2649.57143*), summer-spring (277.32514*) and fall - spring (674.05143 *).

  - For the sodium content in milk, significant differences were found in the mean values at the level of 0.05. The differences are significant in the spring-winter seasons (112.52857*).

5. Based on the mean values of heavy metals and macronutrients in the feed for selected locations, we concluded the following:
   - For the content of copper (Cu) the lowest value is registered in Janciste 1.639 mg / kg, while the highest value is determined in Toplice 17.010 mg / kg. As for the mean of copper calculated from all locations, it is 4.360 mg / kg. The cadmium content is at least present in the samples of feed from Janciste 0.968 µg / kg / 0.000968 mg / kg. The highest concentration of this heavy metal was registered in the samples from Bogovinje 11,966 µg / kg / 0.011966 mg / kg and Toplice 11.498 µg / kg / 0.011498 mg / kg. The mean value of cadmium in feed from all locations was 5.648 µg / kg / 0.005648 mg / kg.
   - The lead content is lowest in Bogovinje 15,239 µg / kg / 0.015239 mg / kg, while the highest value is registered in Toplice 63.603 µg / kg / 0.063603 mg / kg. The mean value for lead calculated from all locations is 34.017 µg / kg / 0.034017 mg / kg.
   - The highest value for manganese is registered in Toplice 98.298 mg / kg, while the lowest in Jegunovce 4.037 mg / kg. The average value of manganese from all locations is 22.807 mg / kg.
   - The lowest nickel content was determined in Toplice 23.357 µg / kg / 0.023357 mg / kg, and the highest value was registered in Poroj 198.637 µg / kg / 0.198637 mg / kg. The mean value of nickel from all locations is 73.876 µg / kg / 0.073876 mg / kg.
   - Zinc is at least present in the samples from Negotino 16.157 mg / kg, while it is most present in the feed from Toplice 100.693 mg / kg. As for the mean value of zinc from all locations, it is 32.412 mg / kg.
   - The lowest content of potassium was determined in Jegunovce 2700.00 mg / kg, and the highest value shows 4480.00 mg / kg, in the samples of the feed taken from the location Toplice. The average value of potassium from all locations is 3382.857 mg / kg.
   - Calcium shows the lowest value in the samples from Toplice 7050.00 mg / kg, and the highest content is present in the samples from Poroj 14400.00 mg / kg. Otherwise, the mean value of calcium from all selected locations is 10635.710 mg / kg.
   - The highest magnesium content is in Toplice 2380.00 mg / kg while the lowest in the feed from Negotino 830.00 mg / kg.
   - The mean sodium value from all selected sites was 658.571 mg / kg. Sodium shows the lowest value in the feed from Negotino 70.00 mg

/ kg, and the highest content is present in the samples from Toplice 1680.00 mg / kg.

6. According to the obtained results for the correlation between the content of heavy metals in raw milk and feed, we came to the following conclusions:
    - There is a very weak positive correlation between copper in feed and milk (r = 0.125). There is no statistical significance between the values of copper in the feed and milk. Between cadmium in feed and milk there is a weak positive correlation (r = 0.169). The correlation is significant at the level of 0.05 (two-way correlation).
    - Regarding the correlation with the element lead, it can be determined that there is a very weak negative correlation between lead in feed and milk (r = - 0.062).
    - There is no statistical significance between the values of lead in feed and milk.
    - There is a very weak negative correlation (r = - 0.017) between manganese in feed and milk, and there is no statistical significance.
    - Among the nickel content in feed and milk there is a very weak positive correlation (r = 0.008). There is no statistical significance between the given values.
    - For the element zinc it can be determined that there is a weak positive correlation between zinc in feed and milk (r = 0.1694). There is no statistical significance between the values.
    - From the statistical analysis of the macronutrients it can be determined that there is a very weak negative correlation between potassium, calcium and magnesium in feed and milk (r = - 0.017; -0.075; -0.084). There is no statistical significance between the values of the selected elements in the feed and milk.
    - From the obtained results it can be determined that there is a weak positive correlation between sodium in feed and milk (r = 0.169). The correlation is significant at the level of 0.05.
7. Based on the obtained results for the incidence of diseases in the region, and the assumption that heavy metals are a potential factor for the occurrence of diseases in the population, given that in our research the selected heavy metals showed normal values with the exception of lead which had a minimal increase above the WHO / FAO values, we believe that more thorough and extensive research is needed on this issue. At the same time, it is necessary to take appropriate measures to prevent contamination of milk with heavy metals, as well as raising environmental awareness as well as the awareness of consuming safe products in order to protect the health of consumers in the region and in the country in general.

RECOMMENDATIONS

1. Training of farmers in order to improve the quality and safety of raw milk, through improved farm hygiene, the process of milking and storage of milk as well as changing the breeding system in a timely manner (to leave the tied system of keeping dairy cows).
2. Giving recommendations for prevention of farm construction and livestock keeping near a source of pollution, as well as agricultural areas for feed production. In our case, the lead content compared between the locations was the highest in the milk from the farm close to the industrial capacity Jugohrom, at the location Jegunovce, as well as the locations Bogovinje and Toplice which are located close to the highway E-65.
3. Preferring more frequent analysis and quality control of feed and milk for the presence of heavy metals and other contaminants.
4. Raising the awareness of farmers and the general public about the importance of food safety, environmental protection and preservation of public health.

REFERENCES

Ayar, A., Sert, D., & Akm, N. (2009). The trace metal levels in milk and dairy products consumed in middle Anatolia-Turkey. *Environmental Monitoring and Assessment, 152*(1-4), 1–12. doi:10.100710661-008-0291-9 PMID:18478348

Bogut, I. (2000). Concentrations of Hg, Pb, Cd and As in meat of fish-pond carp (Cyprinus carpio). *Agriculuture, 6*, 123–125.

Buldini, P. L., Cavalli, S., & Sharma, J. L. (2002). Matrix removal for the ion chromatographic determination of some trace elements in milk. *Microchemical Journal, 72*(3), 277–284. doi:10.1016/S0026-265X(02)00039-5

Ghindini, S., Zanardi, E., & Battaglia, A. (2005). Comparison of contaminat and residue levels in organic and conventional milk and meat products from Northern Italy. *Food Additives and Contaminants, 22*(1), 9–14. doi:10.1080/02652030400027995 PMID:15895606

Grue, C. E., Gibert, P. E., & Seeley, M. E. (1997). Neurophysiological and behavioral changes in non-target wildlife exposed to organophosphate and carbamate pesticides: Thermoregulation, food consumption, and reproduction. *American Zoologist, 37*(4), 369–388. doi:10.1093/icb/37.4.369

Licata, P., Trombetta, D., Cristani, M., Giofre, F., Martino, D., Calo, M., & Niccari, F. (2004). Levels of toxic and essential metals in samples of bovine milk from various dairy farms in Calabria Italy. *Environment International*, *30*(1), 1–6. doi:10.1016/S0160-4120(03)00139-9 PMID:14664858

Lopez, A. M. (2002). Interactions between toxic and essential trace metals in cattle from a region with low levels of pollution. *Archives of Environmental Contamination and Toxicology*, *42*, 165–172. doi:10.100700244-001-0012-7 PMID:11815807

Mehri, H. (2004). *Heavy metal contamination of milk, veterinary* [PhD thesis]. University of Tehran.

Mustafa, S. K. (2020). Polyphenols more than an Antioxidant: Role and Scope. *Journal of Pure & Applied Microbiology*, *14*(1), 47–61. doi:10.22207/JPAM.14.1.08

Nwude, D. O., Okoye, P. A. C., & Babayemi, J. O. (2010). Blood heavy metal levels in cows at slaughter at Awka abattoir. *International Journal of Dairy Science*, *5*(4), 264–270. doi:10.3923/ijds.2010.264.270

Pavlovic, I., Sikiric, M., Havranek, L., Plavljanic, N., & Brajenovic, N. (2004). Lead and cadmium levels in raw cow's milk from anindustrialised Croatian region determined by electrothermal atomic absorption spectrometry. *Czech Journal of Animal Science*, *49*(4), 164–168. doi:10.17221/4295-CJAS

Rocha, C. A., Sousa, F. W., Zanella, M. E., Oliveira, A. G., Nascimento, R. F., Souza, O. V., Cajazeiras, I. M. P., Lima, J. L. R., & Cavalcante, R. M. (2017). Environmental Quality Assessment in Areas Used for Physical Activity and Recreation in a City Affected by Intense Urban Expansion (Fortaleza-CE, Brazil): Implications for Public Health Policy. *Exposure and Health*, *9*(3), 169–182. doi:10.100712403-016-0230-x

Compilation of References

Agosti, S., Casalino, L., Bertero, G., Barsotti, A., Brunelli, C., & Morelloni, S. (2012). A dangerous fruit juice. *The American Journal of Emergency Medicine, 30*(1), 248.

Akoko, J. (2020). Serological and molecular evidence of Brucella species in the rapidly growing pig sector in Kenya. *BioMed Central, 16*(1), 1-7.

Alissa, E. M. (2014). Medicinal Herbs and Therapeutic Drugs Interactions. *Therapeutic Drug Monitoring, 36*(4), 413–422. doi:10.1097/FTD.0000000000000035 PMID:24452064

Allikmets, K. (2007). Aliskiren--An orally active renin inhibitor. Review of pharmacology, pharmacodynamics, kinetics, and clinical potential in the treatment of hypertension. *Vascular Health and Risk Management, 3*(6), 809–815.

Aloia, D. (2016). Medical Rhymes. *Nyamhistorymed.* https://nyamcenterforhistory.org/2016/04/21/medical-rhymes/

Amadi, C. N., & Mgbahurike, A. A. (2018). Selected food/herb–drug interactions: Mechanisms and clinical relevance. *American Journal of Therapeutics, 25*(4), e423–e433. doi:10.1097/MJT.0000000000000705 PMID:29232282

Anlamlert, W., Sermsappasuk, P., Yokubol, D., & Jones, S. (2015). Pomelo enhances cyclosporine bioavailability in healthy male Thai volunteers. *Journal of Clinical Pharmacology, 55*(4), 377–383. doi:10.1002/jcph.430 PMID:25408261

Anonymous. (2012). Fluoroquinolones. In *LiverTox: Clinical and Research Information on Drug-Induced Liver Injury*. National Institute of Diabetes and Digestive and Kidney Diseases. https://www.ncbi.nlm.nih.gov/books/NBK547840/

Anonymous. (2022a). *Detroit Wayne County Health Authority*. Fostering Success Michigan. http://fosteringsuccessmichigan.com/network/detroit-wayne-county-health-authority

Anonymous. (2022b). *Frisco Baseball & Softball Association.* FBSA. https://fbsa.org/content/9226/FAQ

Anonymous. (2022c). *NADIS - National Animal Disease Information Service.* NADIS. https://www.nadis.org.uk/about/

Anonymous. (2022d). *Treasure Valley Orchid Society*. Treasure Valley. http://www.treasurevalleyorchidsociety.org/

Asher, G. N., Corbett, A. H., & Hawke, R. L. (2017). Common Herbal Dietary Supplement-Drug Interactions. *American Family Physician*, *96*(2), 101–107. PMID:28762712

Azevedo-Barbosa, H., Dias, D. F., Franco, L. L., Hawkes, J. A., & Carvalho, D. T. (2020). From Antibacterial to Antitumour Agents: A Brief Review on The Chemical and Medicinal Aspects of Sulfonamides. *Mini-Reviews in Medicinal Chemistry*, *20*(19), 2052–2066. doi:10.2174/1389557520666200905125738 PMID:32888265

Bailey, D., Spence, J., Munoz, C., & Arnold, J. (1991). Interaction of citrus juices with felodipine and nifedipine. *Lancet*, *337*(8736), 268–269. doi:10.1016/0140-6736(91)90872-M PMID:1671113

Bajraktari, G., Koltai, M. S., Ademaj, F., Rexhepaj, N., Qirko, S., Ndrepepa, G., & Elezi, S. (2006). Relationship between insulin resistance and left ventricular diastolic dysfunction in patients with impaired glucose tolerance and type 2 diabetes. *International Journal of Cardiology*, *110*(2), 206–211. doi:10.1016/j.ijcard.2005.08.033 PMID:16297997

Banno, K. (2012). Progestin therapy for endometrial cancer: The potential of fourth-generation progestin [Review]. *International Journal of Oncology*, *40*(6), 1755–1762. doi:10.3892/ijo.2012.1384 PMID:22366992

Bano, G., Raina, R., Zutshi, U., Bedi, K., Johri, R., & Sharma, S. (1991). Effect of piperine on bioavailability and pharmacokinetics of propranolol and theophylline in healthy volunteers. *European Journal of Clinical Pharmacology*, *41*(6), 615–617. doi:10.1007/BF00314996 PMID:1815977

Barreira, P., Basilico, M., & Bolotnyy, V. J. H. U. (2018). Graduate student mental health: Lessons from American economics departments. *NIH*.

Bazzie, K. L., Witmer, D. R., Pinto, B., Bush, C., Clark, J., & Deffenbaugh, J. Jr. (2006). National survey of dietary supplement policies in acute care facilities. *American Journal of Health-System Pharmacy*, *63*(1), 65–70. doi:10.2146/ajhp050106 PMID:16373467

Beaulieu, M., Nadeau, A., Lacourcière, Y., & Cléroux, J. (1993). Post-exercise reduction in blood pressure in hypertensive subjects: Effects of angiotensin converting enzyme inhibition. *British Journal of Clinical Pharmacology*, *36*(4), 331–338. doi:10.1111/j.1365-2125.1993.tb00372.x PMID:12959311

Becquemont, L., Verstuyft, C., Kerb, R., Brinkmann, U., Lebot, M., Jaillon, P., & Funck-Brentano, C. (2001). Effect of grapefruit juice on digoxin pharmacokinetics in humans. *Clinical Pharmacology and Therapeutics*, *70*(4), 311–316. doi:10.1016/S0009-9236(01)13478-8 PMID:11673746

Bedan, M., Grimm, D., Wehland, M., Simonsen, U., Infanger, M., & Krüger, M. (2018). A Focus on Macitentan in the Treatment of Pulmonary Arterial Hypertension. *Basic & Clinical Pharmacology & Toxicology*, *123*(2), 103–113. doi:10.1111/bcpt.13033 PMID:29719121

Beik, A., Joukar, S., & Najafipour, H. (2020). A review on plants and herbal components with antiarrhythmic activities and their interaction with current cardiac drugs. *Journal of Traditional and Complementary Medicine*, *10*(3), 275–287. doi:10.1016/j.jtcme.2020.03.002 PMID:32670823

Belda, J., Margarit, G., Martinez, C., Bellido-Casado, J., Casan, P., Torrejon, M., Brufal, M., Rodriguez-Jerez, F., & Sanchis, J. (2007). Anti-inflammatory effects of high-dose inhaled fluticasone versus oral prednisone in asthma exacerbations. *The European Respiratory Journal*, *30*(6), 1143–1149. doi:10.1183/09031936.00050306 PMID:17690122

Berk, M., Dean, O., Drexhage, H., McNeil, J. J., Moylan, S., O'Neil, A., Davey, C. G., Sanna, L., & Maes, M. (2013). Aspirin: A review of its neurobiological properties and therapeutic potential for mental illness. *BMC Medicine*, *11*(1), 1–17. doi:10.1186/1741-7015-11-74 PMID:23506529

Berman, B.M. (2001). Complementary medicine and medical education. *BMJ*, *322*(7279), 121–122.

Bertram, G. K. (2018). *Basic & clinical pharmacology* (14th ed.). McGraw-Hill Education.

Bhandari, P. (2018). Adrenergic Drugs. In Pharmacology for Medical Undergraduates (pp. 67–67). Jaypee Brothers Medical Publishers (P) Ltd. doi:10.5005/jp/books/14244_9

Bhardwaj, R. K., Glaeser, H., Becquemont, L., Klotz, U., Gupta, S. K., & Fromm, M. F. (2002). Piperine, a major constituent of black pepper, inhibits human P-glycoprotein and CYP3A4. *The Journal of Pharmacology and Experimental Therapeutics*, *302*(2), 645–650. doi:10.1124/jpet.102.034728 PMID:12130727

Bian, H., Bian, Y., Li, J., Xu, S., Shao, X., Li, J., & Jiang, B. (2020, March 1). A simple hand mnemonic for teaching the cardiac cycle. *Advances in Physiology Education*, *44*(1), 21–25. doi:10.1152/advan.00059.2019 PMID:31821034

Binks, A.P., (2021). Changing medical education, overnight: the curricular response to COVID-19 of nine medical schools. *NIH, 33*(3), p. 334-342.

Bistrup, C., Nielsen, F. T., Jeppesen, U. E., & Dieperink, H. (2001). Effect of grapefruit juice on Sandimmun Neoral® absorption among stable renal allograft recipients. *Nephrology, Dialysis, Transplantation*, *16*(2), 373–377. doi:10.1093/ndt/16.2.373 PMID:11158415

Borovac, J. A. (2016). Side effects of a dopamine agonist therapy for Parkinson's disease: a mini-review of clinical pharmacology. *The Yale Journal of Biology and Medicine, 89*(1), 37–47.

Bos, A., Kruse, F.M., & Jeurissen, P. (2020). *For-profit nursing homes in the Netherlands: what factors explain their rise? NIH,* (4), p. 431-443.

Bosch, N. A., Cimini, J., & Walkey, A. J. (2018). Atrial Fibrillation in the ICU. *Chest*, *154*(6), 1424–1434. doi:10.1016/j.chest.2018.03.040 PMID:29627355

Brosch, T., Scherer, K. R., Grandjean, D., & Sander, D. (2013). The impact of emotion on perception, attention, memory, and decision-making. *Swiss Medical Weekly*, *143*, w13786. doi:10.4414mw.2013.13786 PMID:23740562

Brown, C., Taniguchi, G., & Yip, K. (1989). The monoamine oxidase inhibitor—Tyramine interaction. *Journal of Clinical Pharmacology*, *29*(6), 529–532. doi:10.1002/j.1552-4604.1989.tb03376.x PMID:2666453

Brunton, L. L., Chabner, B. A., & Knollmann, B. C. (2011). The Pharmacological basis of Therapeutics. In L. L. Brunton, B. A. Chabner, & B. C. Knollmann (Eds.), *The pharmacological basis of Therapeutics*. Elsevier. https://linkinghub.elsevier.com/retrieve/pii/B9780323481106000302

Brunton, L., Knollmann, B., & Hilal-Dandan, R. (2017). *Goodman and Gilman's, The Pharmacological Basis of Therapeutics* (13th ed.). McGraw-Hill.

Busse, W. W., Mcgill, K. A., & Horwitz, R. J. (1999). Leukotriene pathway inhibitors in asthma and chronic obstructive pulmonary disease. *Clinical and Experimental Allergy*, *29*(2), 110–115. doi:10.1046/j.1365-2222.1999.00019.x PMID:10421833

Caterina, P., Antonello, D. P., Chiara, G., Chiara, C., Giacomo, L., & Antonio, S. (2013). Pharmacokinetic drug-drug interaction and their implication in clinical management. *Journal of Research in Medical Sciences*, *18*, 601–610. PMID:24516494

Catto, G., Cork, N., & Williams, G. (2014). Should medical students be taught alternative medicine? *British Medical Journal*, *348*(g2417), 1–3. doi:10.1136/bmj.g2417 PMID:24682533

Chan, W. (2018). President's Whitepaper Project: Global Literacy at the University of Maryland, Baltimore. University of Maryland.

Chan, L. N. (2013). Drug-nutrient interactions. *Journal of Parenteral and Enteral Nutrition*, *37*(4), 450–459. doi:10.1177/0148607113488799 PMID:23674575

Cheng, Y.-Y., Hsieh, C.-H., & Tsai, T.-H. (2018). Concurrent administration of anticancer chemotherapy drug and herbal medicine on the perspective of pharmacokinetics. *Yao Wu Shi Pin Fen Xi*, *26*(2), S88–S95 . https://doi.org/10.1016/j.jfda.2018.01.003.

Chen, H. H., & Burnett, J. C. Jr. (1999). The Natriuretic Peptides in Heart Failure: Diagnostic and Therapeutic Potentials. *Proceedings of the Association of American Physicians*, *111*(5), 406–416. doi:10.1111/paa.1999.111.5.406 PMID:10519161

Chen, M., Zhou, S. Y., Fabriaga, E., Zhang, P. H., & Zhou, Q. (2018). Food-drug interactions precipitated by fruit juices other than grapefruit juice: An update review. *Yao Wu Shi Pin Fen Xi*, *26*(2S), S61–S71 . https://doi.org/10.1016/j.jfda.2018.01.009]. .

Chen, T. (2017). Hepatotoxicity of Herbal Supplements Mediated by Modulation of Cytochrome P450. *International Journal of Molecular Sciences*, *18*(11), 2353. https://doi.org/10.3390/ijms18112353

Chen, X. W., Sneed, K. B., Pan, S. Y., Cao, C., Kanwar, J. R., Chew, H., & Zhou, S. F. (2012). Herb-drug interactions and mechanistic and clinical considerations. *Current Drug Metabolism*, *13*(5), 640–651. doi:10.2174/1389200211209050640 PMID:22292789

Choi, J. H., & Ko, C. M. (2017). Food and drug interactions. *Journal of Lifestyle Medicine*, *7*(1), 1–9. doi:10.15280/jlm.2017.7.1.1 PMID:28261555

Chopra, I., & Roberts, M. (2001). Tetracycline Antibiotics: Mode of Action, Applications, Molecular Biology, and Epidemiology of Bacterial Resistance. *Microbiology and Molecular Biology Reviews*, *65*(2), 232–260. doi:10.1128/MMBR.65.2.232-260.2001 PMID:11381101

Christensen, C. M., Morris, R. S., Kapsandoy, S. C., Archer, M., Kuang, J., Shane-McWhorter, L., Bray, B. E., & Zeng-Treitler, Q. (2017). Patient needs and preferences for herb-drug-disease interaction alerts: a structured interview. *BMC Complementary and Alternative Medicine, 17*, 272. doi:1630-6 doi:10.1186/s12906-017-

Cirigliano, M. M. (2013). Musical mnemonics in health science: A first look. *Medical Teacher*, *35*(3), e1020–e1026. https://doi.org/10.3109/0142159X.2012.733042

Colombo, D., Lunardon, L., & Bellia, G. (2014). Cyclosporine and Herbal Supplement Interactions. *Journal of Toxicology*, *2014*, 145325. https://doi.org/10.1155/2014/145325.

Colovic, M. B., Krstic, D. Z., Lazarevic-Pasti, T. D., Bondzic, A. M., & Vasic, V. M. (2013). Acetylcholinesterase Inhibitors: Pharmacology and Toxicology. *Current Neuropharmacology*, *11*(3), 315–335. doi:10.2174/1570159X11311030006 PMID:24179466

Committee for Human Medicinal Products. (2012). *Guideline on the investigation of drug interactions.* European Medicines Agency, Science Medicines Health.

Costache, I. I., Miron, A., Hăncianu, M., Aursulesei, V., Costache, A. D., & Aprotosoaie, A. C. (2019). Pharmacokinetic Interactions between Cardiovascular Medicines and Plant Products. *Cardiovascular Therapeutics*, *9402781*, 1–19. doi:10.1155/2019/9402781 PMID:32089733

Cree, W. J. (1944) In memoriam: Hugo Erichsen M.D. *Detroit Medical News, 36*(12), 9.

Crowell-Davis, S. L. (2019). Tricyclic Antidepressants. In *Veterinary Psychopharmacology* (pp. 231–256). Wiley. doi:10.1002/9781119226253.ch16

Custodio, J. M., Wu, C.-Y., & Benet, L. Z. (2008). Predicting drug disposition, absorption/elimination/transporter interplay and the role of food on drug absorption. *Advanced Drug Delivery Reviews*, *60*(6), 717–733. doi:10.1016/j.addr.2007.08.043 PMID:18199522

Dai, L., Liu, A., Zhang, H., Wu, H., Zhang, T., Su, B., Shao, Y., Li, J., Ye, J., Scott, S. R., Mahajan, S. D., Schwartz, S. A., Yu, H., & Sun, L. (2019). Impact of Lopinavir/Ritonavir and Efavirenz-Based Antiretroviral Therapy on the Lipid Profile of Chinese HIV/AIDS Treatment-Naïve Patients in Beijing: A Retrospective Study. *Current HIV Research*, *17*(5), 324–334. doi:10.2174/1570162X17666191025115508 PMID:31654514

Dasgupta, A. (2008). Drug–Herb and Drug–Food Interactions. Handbook of Drug Monitoring Methods, 235-261.

Dasgupta, A., Kidd, L., Poindexter, B. J., & Bick, R. J. (2010). Interference of Hawthorn on serum digoxin measurements by immunoassays and pharmacodynamic interaction with digoxin. *Archives of Pathology & Laboratory Medicine, 134*(8), 1188–1192. doi:10.5858/2009-0404-OA.1 PMID:20670141

David, M. N. V., & Shetty, M. (2021). Digoxin. *StatPearls [Internet]. Treasure Island (FL): StatPearls Publishing.* https://www.ncbi.nlm.nih.gov/books/NBK556025/

Davis, S. A., Feldman, S. R., & Taylor, S. L. (2014). Use of St. John's Wort in potentially dangerous combinations. *Journal of Alternative and Complementary Medicine (New York, N.Y.), 20*(7), 578–579. doi:10.1089/acm.2013.0216 PMID:24956073

De Castro, W. V., Mertens-Talcott, S., Derendorf, H., & Butterweck, V. (2007). Grapefruit juice–drug interactions: Grapefruit juice and its components inhibit P-glycoprotein (ABCB1) mediated transport of talinolol in Caco-2 cells. *Journal of Pharmaceutical Sciences, 96*(10), 2808–2817. doi:10.1002/jps.20975 PMID:17542018

de Lemos, M. L., Hamata, L., Jennings, S., & Leduc, T. (2007). Interaction between mercaptopurine and milk. *Journal of Oncology Pharmacy Practice, 13*(4), 237–240. doi:10.1177/1078155207080802 PMID:18045784

de Lima Toccafondo Vieira, M., & Huang, S. M. (2012). Botanical-drug interactions: A scientific perspective. *Planta Medica, 78*(13), 1400–1415. doi:10.1055-0032-1315145 PMID:22864989

Debnath. S., Tejovathi. R., Babu. N. & Kumar. T. H. H (2017). An Overview on Food & Drug Interactions. *Pharma Times, 49*, 4.

Dennen, V.P. (2022). Supporting new online instructors and engaging remote learners during COVID-19: a distributed team teaching approach. *NIH, 54*(sup1), S182-S202.

Djamshidian, A., & Poewe, W. (2016). Apomorphine and levodopa in Parkinson's disease: Two revolutionary drugs from the 1950's. *Parkinsonism & Related Disorders, 33*, S9–S12. doi:10.1016/j.parkreldis.2016.12.004 PMID:28012951

Dobos, G., & Tao, I. (2011). The model of western integrative medicine: The role of Chinese medicine. *Chinese Journal of Integrative Medicine, 17*(1), 11–20. https://doi.org/10.1007/s11655-011-0601-x. .

Doostdar, H., Burke, M. D., & Mayer, R. T. (2000). Bioflavonoids: Selective substrates and inhibitors for cytochrome P450 CYP1A and CYP1B1. *Toxicology, 1*(144), 31–38. doi:10.1016/S0300-483X(99)00215-2 PMID:10781868

Dresser, G. K., Kim, R. B., & Bailey, D. G. (2005). Effect of grapefruit juice volume on the reduction of fexofenadine bioavailability: Possible role of organic anion transporting polypeptides. *Clinical Pharmacology and Therapeutics, 77*(3), 170–177. doi:10.1016/j.clpt.2004.10.005 PMID:15735611

Dürr, D. (2000). St John's Wort induces intestinal P-glycoprotein/MDR1 and intestinal and hepatic CYP3A4. *Clinical Pharmacology and Therapeutics*, *68*(6), 598–604. doi:10.1067/mcp.2000.112240 PMID:11180019

Edwards, N. (2023). *Research Education Program for Underrepresented Minority Students: Students' Perception of Academic Enrichment and Research Activities.* NIH.

Egashira, K., Fukuda, E., Onga, T., Yogi, Y., Matsuya, F., Koyabu, N., Ohtani, H., & Sawada, Y. (2003). Pomelo-induced increase in the blood level of tacrolimus in a renal transplant patient. *Transplantation*, *75*(7), 1057. doi:10.1097/01.TP.0000058545.35041.BE PMID:12698101

Ekor, M. (2014). The growing use of herbal medicines: issues relating to adverse reactions and challenges in monitoring safety. *Frontiers in Pharmacology, 4*. doi:10.3389/fphar.2013.00177

Elliott, R. Camacho, E. Campbell, F. Jankovic, D. Martyn St. James, M. Kaltenthaler, E. Wong, R. Sculpher, M. J., & Faria, R. (2018). Prevalence and Economic Burden of Medication Errors in the NHS in England. In *Rapid Evidence Synthesis and Economic Analysis of the Prevalence and Burden of Medication Error in the UK.* Policy Research Unit in Economic Evaluation of Health and Care Interventions Universities of Sheffield and York, Manchester, UK.

Erichsen, H., St. Louis, M. O., & Chambers, J. H. (1884) Medical Rhymes.

Eyler, R. F., & Shvets, K. (2019). Clinical Pharmacology of Antibiotics. *Clinical Journal of the American Society of Nephrology; CJASN*, *14*(7), 1080–1090. https://doi.org/10.2215/CJN.08140718

Ezmed. (2022, January 20). *Cranial Nerves MADE EASY: Mnemonic & Tricks for Their Names & Function.* [Video] YouTube. https://www.youtube.com/watch?v=fELPJIjC7E4

Fagan, T. C., Walle, T., Oexmann, M. J., Walle, U. K., Bai, S. A., & Gaffney, T. E. (1987). Increased clearance of propranolol and theophylline by high-protein compared with high-carbohydrate diet. *Clinical Pharmacology and Therapeutics*, *41*(4), 402–406. doi:10.1038/clpt.1987.48 PMID:3829577

Fairweather-Tait, S., Hickson, K., McGaw, B., & Reid, M. (1994). Orange juice enhances aluminium absorption from antacid preparation. *European Journal of Clinical Nutrition*, *48*(1), 71–73. PMID:8200332

Farzam, K., & Jan, A. (2018). Drugs in Sport. In D. R. Mottram & N. Chester (Eds.), Drugs in Sport (7th ed.). Routledge. doi:10.4324/9781315222790

Fasinu, P. S., & Rapp, G. K. (2019). Herbal Interaction with Chemotherapeutic Drugs—A Focus on Clinically Significant Findings. *Frontiers in Oncology, 9*. doi:10.3389/fonc.2019.01356

Fasinu , P. S., Bouic, P. J., & Rosenkranz, B. (2012). An overview of the evidence and mechanisms of herb–drug interactions. *Front. Pharmacol, 3*(69).

Fasinu, P. S., Bouic, P. J., & Rosenkranz, B. (2012). An overview of the evidence and mechanisms of herb-drug interactions. *Frontiers in Pharmacology*, *3*, 69. doi:10.3389/fphar.2012.00069 PMID:22557968

Food and Drug Administration. (2016, December). *Botanical Drug Development: Guidance for Industry*. FDA. https://www.fda.gov/regulatory-information/search-fda-guidance-documents/botanical-drug-development-guidance-industry from https://www.who.int/news-room/factsheets/detail/c ardiovascular-diseases-cvds)

Freeland, B., & Farber, M. S. (2016). A Review of Insulin for the Treatment of Diabetes Mellitus. *Home Healthcare Now*, *34*(8), 416–423. doi:10.1097/NHH.0000000000000446 PMID:27580280

Frenkel, M., Ben-Arye, E. & Hermoni, D. (2004). An approach to educating family practice residents and family physicians about complementary and alternative medicine Complement. *Ther. Med.*, *12*(2-3), 118-25.

Fugh-Berman, A. (2000). Herb-drug interactions. *Lancet*, *355*(9198), 134–138. doi:10.1016/S0140-6736(99)06457-0 PMID:10675182

Fuhr, U., Müller-Peltzer, H., Kern, R., Lopez-Rojas, P., Jünemann, M., Harder, S., & Staib, H. A. (2002). Effects of grapefruit juice and smoking on verapamil concentrations in steady state. *European Journal of Clinical Pharmacology*, *58*(1), 45–53. doi:10.100700228-002-0436-7 PMID:11956673

Fujita, K.-i. (2004). Food-drug interactions via human cytochrome P450 3A (CYP3A). *Drug Metabolism and Drug Interactions*, *20*(4), 195–218. doi:10.1515/DMDI.2004.20.4.195 PMID:15663291

Gabay, M., & Spencer, S. H. (2021). Chronic Conditions and Public Health. *PSAP*, *3*. https://www.accp.com/docs/bookstore/psap/p2021b3_sample.pdf

Ganesan, K., Rana, M. B. M., & Sultan, S. (2022). Oral Hypoglycemic Medications. In *StatPearls*. StatPearls Publishing. https://www.ncbi.nlm.nih.gov/books/NBK482386/

Gardiner, P., Phillips, R. S., & Shaughnessy, A. F. (2008). Herbal and dietary supplement-drug interactions in patients with chronic illnesses. *American Family Physician*, *77*(1), 73–78. PMID:18236826

Garg, S. K., Kumar, N., Bhargava, V. K., & Prabhakar, S. K. (1998). Effect of grapefruit juice on carbamazepine bioavailability in patients with epilepsy. *Clinical Pharmacology and Therapeutics*, *64*(3), 286–288. doi:10.1016/S0009-9236(98)90177-1 PMID:9757152

Gayatri, D. (2021). Quality of life of cancer patients at palliative care units in developing countries: systematic review of the published literature. *NIH*, *30*(2), 315-343.

Geisen, S. M., & Sturla, S. J. (2019). Can Foods or Herbs Alter the Bioavailability of Chemotherapy Drugs? *ACS Pharmacology & Translational Science*, *2*(2), 143–146. doi:10.1021/acsptsci.9b00007

Genser, D. (2008). Food and drug interaction: Consequences for the nutrition/health status. *Annals of Nutrition & Metabolism*, *52*(Suppl. 1), 29–32. doi:10.1159/000115345 PMID:18382075

Giovannitti, J. A. Jr, Thoms, S. M., & Crawford, J. J. (2015). Alpha-2 Adrenergic Receptor Agonists: A Review of Current Clinical Applications. *Anesthesia Progress*, *62*(1), 31–38. doi:10.2344/0003-3006-62.1.31 PMID:25849473

Glenn Schellenberg, E. (2011). Music lessons, emotional intelligence, and IQ. *Music Perception*, *29*(2), 185–194.

Goey, A. K. L., Meijerman, I., Rosing, H., Marchetti, S., Mergui-Roelvink, M., Keessen, M., Burgers, J. A., Beijnen, J. H., & Schellens, J. H. M. (2013). The Effect of St John's Wort on the Pharmacokinetics of Docetaxel. [Retrieved from https://doi.org/10.1007/s40262-013-0102-5]. *Clinical Pharmacokinetics*, *53*(1), 103–110.

Gray, A.C. (2022). *An examination of the prevalence, impact, experiences and perceptions of learning and health technologies on students, academics and educational leaders in complementary medicine education institutions: A mixed method study of two institutions, one in Australia and one in the US*. University of Technology Sydney.

Gray, A. C., Steel, A., & Adams, J. (2019). A critical integrative review of complementary medicine education research: Key issues and empirical gaps. *BMC Complementary and Alternative Medicine*, *19*(1), 73. doi:10.118612906-019-2466-z PMID:30894151

Grenier, J., Fradette, C., Morelli, G., Merritt, G. J., Vranderick, M., & Ducharme, M. P. (2006). Pomelo juice, but not cranberry juice, affects the pharmacokinetics of cyclosporine in humans. *Clinical Pharmacology and Therapeutics*, *79*(3), 255–262. doi:10.1016/j.clpt.2005.11.010 PMID:16513449

Grimstein, M., & Huang, S. M. (2018). A regulatory science viewpoint on botanical-drug interactions. *Yao Wu Shi Pin Fen Xi*, *26*(2), 12–25. doi:10.1016/j.jfda.2018.01.013 PMID:29703380

Gubbins, P. O., McConnell, S. A., Gurley, B. J., Fincher, T. K., Franks, A. M., Williams, D. K., Penzak, S. R., & Saccente, M. (2004). Influence of grapefruit juice on the systemic availability of itraconazole oral solution in healthy adult volunteers. *Pharmacotherapy: The Journal of Human Pharmacology and Drug Therapy*, *24*(4), 460–467. doi:10.1592/phco.24.5.460.33350 PMID:15098799

Guo, J., Xuan, Z. Y., & Xie, Y. (2020). Problems and considerations in pharmaceutical researches of new traditional Chinese medicine. *Chinese Traditional and Herbal Drugs*, *51*(8), 2267–2272.

Gupta, R. C., Chang, D., Nammi, S., Bensoussan, A., Bilinski, K., & Roufogalis, B. D. (2017). Interactions between antidiabetic drugs and herbs: An overview of mechanisms of action and clinical implications. *Diabetology & Metabolic Syndrome*, *9*(1). https://doi.org/10.1186/s13098-017-0254-9]. .

Gurley, B. J., & Hagan, D. W. (2003). Herbal and dietary supplement interactions with drugs. In J. J. Wolfe (Ed.), *Hand book of food-drug Interactions* (pp. 259–293). CRC Press.

Hamoda, H., Panay, N., Pedder, H., Arya, R., & Savvas, M. (2020). The British Menopause Society & Women's Health Concern 2020 recommendations on hormone replacement therapy in menopausal women. *Post Reproductive Health*, *26*(4), 181–209. doi:10.1177/2053369120957514 PMID:33045914

Hanley, M. J., Cancalon, P., Widmer, W. W., & Greenblatt, D. J. (2011). The effect of grapefruit juice on drug disposition. *Expert Opinion on Drug Metabolism & Toxicology*, *7*(3), 267–286. doi:10.1517/17425255.2011.553189 PMID:21254874

Harder, S., & Graff, J. (2013). Novel oral anticoagulants: Clinical pharmacology, indications and practical considerations. *European Journal of Clinical Pharmacology*, *69*(9), 1617–1633. https://doi.org/10.1007/s00228-013-1510-z.

Hargreaves, D. J., MacDonald, R., & Miell, D. (2018). Musical identities mediate musical development. *Music and music education in people's lives, 1*, 124-142.

Harvey, R. A., Clark, M. A., Finkel, R., Rey, J. A., & Whalen, K. (2011). *Pharmacology (Lippincott's Illustrated Reviews Series)*. Lippincott Williams & Wilkins. https://books.google.com/books/about/Pharmacology.html?id=Y558dgp_PjoC

He, K., Iyer, K. R., Hayes, R. N., Sinz, M. W., Woolf, T. F., & Hollenberg, P. F. (1998). Inactivation of cytochrome P450 3A4 by bergamottin, a component of grapefruit juice. *Chemical Research in Toxicology*, *11*(4), 252–259. doi:10.1021/tx970192k PMID:9548795

Hickok, G., Buchsbaum, B., Humphries, C., & Muftuler, T. (2003). Auditory–motor interaction revealed by fMRI: Speech, music, and working memory in area Spt. *Journal of Cognitive Neuroscience*, *15*(5), 673–682.

Hidaka, M., Okumura, M., Fujita, K.-i., Ogikubo, T., Yamasaki, K., Iwakiri, T., Setoguchi, N., & Arimori, K. (2005). Effects of pomegranate juice on human cytochrome p450 3A (CYP3A) and carbamazepine pharmacokinetics in rats. *Drug Metabolism and Disposition: the Biological Fate of Chemicals*, *33*(5), 644–648. doi:10.1124/dmd.104.002824 PMID:15673597

Hiwale, A., Dhuley, J., & Naik, S. (2002). Effect of co-administration of piperine on pharmacokinetics of beta-lactam antibiotics in rats. *Indian Journal of Experimental Biology*, *40*(3), 277–281. PMID:12635696

Holst, J. & Health, P. (2020). Increasing rural recruitment and retention through rural exposure during undergraduate training: an integrative review. *NIH*, *17*(17): p. 6423.

Hosseini, S. M. (2018, June 1). A useful hand mnemonic to demonstrate ion channel gating. *Advances in Physiology Education*, *42*(2), 321–323. doi:10.1152/advan.00080.2017 PMID:29676617

Huang, S. M., Strong, J. M., Zhang, L., Reynolds, K. S., Nallani, S., Temple, R., & Burckart, G. J. (2008). New era in drug interaction evaluation: US Food and Drug Administration update on CYP enzymes, transporters, and the guidance process. *Journal of Clinical Pharmacology*, *48*(6), 662–670. doi:10.1177/0091270007312153 PMID:18378963

Huppertz, A., Werntz, L., Meid, A. D., Foerster, K. I., Burhenne, J., Czock, D., Mikus, G., & Haefeli, W. E. (2018). Rivaroxaban and macitentan can be co-administered without dose adjustment but the combination of rivaroxaban and St John's wort should be avoided. *British Journal of Clinical Pharmacology*, *84*(12), 2903–2913. https://doi.org/10.1111/bcp.13757.

Huxel, C., Raja, A., & Ollivierre-Lawrence, M. D. (2022). Loop Diuretics. In *StatPearls*. StatPearls Publishing. https://www.ncbi.nlm.nih.gov/books/NBK546656/

Hwang, G.-J. (2020). *Vision, challenges, roles and research issues of Artificial Intelligence in Education*. Elsevier. doi:10.1016/j.caeai.2020.100001

Izzo, A. A. (2012). Interactions between herbs and conventional drugs: Overview of the clinical data. *Medical Principles and Practice*, *21*(5), 404–428. doi:10.1159/000334488 PMID:22236736

Jiang, M., Zhang, C., Cao, H., Chan, K., & Lu, A. (2011). The Role of Chinese Medicine in the Treatment of Chronic Diseases in China. *Planta Medica*, *77*(09), 873–881. https://doi.org/10.1055/s-0030-1270983.

Kalpaklioglu, F., & Baccioglu, A. (2012). Efficacy and Safety of H1-Antihistamines: An Update. *Anti-Inflammatory & Anti-Allergy Agents in Medicinal Chemistry*, *11*(3), 230–237. doi:10.2174/1871523011202030230 PMID:23173575

Kamath, A. V., Yao, M., Zhang, Y., & Chong, S. (2005). Effect of fruit juices on the oral bioavailability of fexofenadine in rats. *Journal of Pharmaceutical Sciences*, *94*(2), 233–239. doi:10.1002/jps.20231 PMID:15570603

Kam, P. C. A., & Liew, S. (2002). Traditional Chinese herbal medicine and anaesthesia. *Anaesthesia*, *57*(11), 1083–1089. https://doi.org/10.1046/j.1365-2044.2002.02823.x.

Kantor, M. (2009). The role of rigorous scientific evaluation in the use and practice of complementary and alternative medicine. *Journal of the American College of Radiology*, *6*(4), 254–262. doi:10.1016/j.jacr.2008.09.012 PMID:19327658

Katzung, B. G. (2015). Basic & Clinical Pharmacology (14th ed.). McGraw Hill.

Kay, G. G., Abou-Donia, M. B., Messer, W. S. Jr, Murphy, D. G., Tsao, J. W., & Ouslander, J. G. (2005). Antimuscarinic Drugs for Overactive Bladder and Their Potential Effects on Cognitive Function in Older Patients. *Journal of the American Geriatrics Society*, *53*(12), 2195–2201. doi:10.1111/j.1532-5415.2005.00537.x PMID:16398909

Kennedy, D. R. (2019). Redesigning a Pharmacology Course to Promote Active Learning. *American Journal of Pharmaceutical Education*, *83*(5), 6782. doi:10.5688/ajpe6782 PMID:31333258

Kim, E. J., Chen, Y., Huang, J. Q., Li, K. M., Razmovski-Naumovski, V., Poon, J., Chan, K., Roufogalis, B. D., McLachlan, A. J., Mo, S. L., Yang, D., Yao, M., Liu, Z., Liu, J., & Li, G. Q. (2013). Evidence-based toxicity evaluation and scheduling of Chinese herbal medicines. *Journal of Ethnopharmacology*, *146*(1), 40–61. doi:10.1016/j.jep.2012.12.027 PMID:23286904

Kim, Y. J. (2017). The Current Studies of Education for a Traditional and Complementary Medicine in Malaysia. *Journal of Evidence-Based Complementary & Alternative Medicine, 22*(4), 531–537. doi:10.1177/2156587217726882 PMID:28853309

Kirby, B., & Unadkat, J. (2007). Grapefruit juice, a glass full of drug interactions? *Clinical Pharmacology and Therapeutics, 81*(5), 631–633. doi:10.1038j.clpt.6100185 PMID:17438537

Koitabashi, Y., Kumai, T., Matsumoto, N., Watanabe, M., Sekine, S., Yanagida, Y., & Kobayashi, S. (2006). Orange juice increased the bioavailability of pravastatin, 3-hydroxy-3-methylglutaryl CoA reductase inhibitor, in rats and healthy human subjects. *Life Sciences, 78*(24), 2852–2859. doi:10.1016/j.lfs.2005.11.006 PMID:16412477

Kondal, A., & Garg, S. (2003). Influence of acidic beverage (Coca-Cola) on pharmacokinetics of ibuprofen in healthy rabbits. *Indian Journal of Experimental Biology, 41*(11), 1322–1324. PMID:15332505

Krasowski, M. D., McGehee, D. S., & Moss, J. (1997). Natural inhibitors of cholinesterases: Implications for adverse drug reactions. *Canadian Journal of Anaesthesia, 44*(5), 525–534. doi:10.1007/BF03011943 PMID:9161749

Kumar, N., Garg, S., & Prabhakar, S. (1999). Lack of pharmacokinetic interaction between grapefruit juice and phenytoin in healthy male volunteers and epileptic patients. *Methods and Findings in Experimental and Clinical Pharmacology, 21*(9), 629–632. PMID:10669910

Kumar-Pal, S. (2002). Complementary and alternative medicine: An overview. *Current Science, 82*(5), 513–524.

Kupferschmidt, H. H., Fattinger, K. E., Ha, H. R., Follath, F., & Krähenbühl, S. (1998). Grapefruit juice enhances the bioavailability of the HIV protease inhibitor saquinavir in man. *British Journal of Clinical Pharmacology, 45*(4), 355–359. doi:10.1046/j.1365-2125.1998.t01-1-00687.x PMID:9578182

Kupferschmidt, H. H., Ha, H. R., Ziegler, W. H., Meier, P. J., & Krähenbühl, S. (1995). Interaction between grapefruit juice and midazolam in humans. *Clinical Pharmacology and Therapeutics, 58*(1), 20–28. doi:10.1016/0009-9236(95)90068-3 PMID:7628179

Lally, J., & MacCabe, J. H. (2015). Antipsychotic medication in schizophrenia: A review. *British Medical Bulletin, 114*(1), 169–179. doi:10.1093/bmb/ldv017 PMID:25957394

Lecture Notes on Pharmacology. (2011). *Department of Medical Sciences, University of Pharmacy* (3rd ed.). Ministry of Health, Union of Myanmar.

Lewis, J. B. Jr, Mulligan, R., & Kraus, N. (2018). The importance of medical mnemonics in medicine. *Pharos., 2018*, 30–35.

Li, W., Li, D., Kuang, H., Feng, X., Ai, W., Wang, Y., Shi, S., Chen, J., & Fan, R. (2020). Berberine increases glucose uptake and intracellular ROS levels by promoting Sirtuin 3 ubiquitination. *Biomedicine & Pharmacotherapy, 121*, 109563. doi:10.1016/j.biopha.2019.109563

Lilja, J. J., Juntti-Patinen, L., & Neuvonen, P. J. (2004). Orange juice substantially reduces the bioavailability of the β-adrenergic–blocking agent celiprolol. *Clinical Pharmacology and Therapeutics*, *75*(3), 184–190. doi:10.1016/j.clpt.2003.11.002 PMID:15001969

Lilja, J. J., Kivistö, K. T., & Neuvonen, P. J. (2000). Duration of effect of grapefruit juice on the pharmacokinetics of the CYP3A4 substrate simvastatin. *Clinical Pharmacology and Therapeutics*, *68*(4), 384–390. doi:10.1067/mcp.2000.110216 PMID:11061578

Lim, X. Y., Chan, J. S. W., Japri, N., Lee, J. C., & Tan, T. Y. C. (2021). Carica papaya L. Leaf: A Systematic Scoping Review on Biological Safety and Herb-Drug Interactions. Evidence-Based Complementary and Alternative Medicine. doi:10.1155/2021/5511221

Lim, J., Chee, S., Wong, W., He, Q., & Lau, T. (2018). Traditional Chinese medicine: Herb-drug interactions with aspirin. *Singapore Medical Journal*, *59*(5), 230–239. https://doi.org/10.11622/smedj.2018051.

Lin, H. W., Tsai, H. H., Yu, I. W., Kumar, A., & Wu, M. P. (2014). Would It Matter to Expose Elderly Patients Who Took Digoxin to Chinese Medications? *Value in Health Regional Issues*, *3*, 211–221. doi:10.1016/j.vhri.2014.04.002 PMID:29702930

Liperoti, R., Vetrano, D. L., Bernabei, R., & Onder, G. (2017). Herbal Medications in Cardiovascular Medicine. *Journal of the American College of Cardiology*, *69*(9), 1188–1199. doi:10.1016/j.jacc.2016.11.078 PMID:28254182

Li, X., Hu, J., Wang, B., Sheng, L., Liu, Z., Yang, S., & Li, Y. (2014). Inhibitory effects of herbal constituents on P-glycoprotein in vitro and in vivo: Herb-drug interactions mediated via P-gp. *Toxicology and Applied Pharmacology*, *275*(2), 163–175. doi:10.1016/j.taap.2013.12.015 PMID:24380838

Li, Y., Jiang, X., Lan, K., Zhang, R., Li, X., & Jiang, Q. (2007). Pharmacokinetic properties of rosuvastatin after single-dose, oral administration in Chinese volunteers: A randomized, open-label, three-way crossover study. *Clinical Therapeutics*, *29*(10), 2194–2203. doi:10.1016/j.clinthera.2007.10.005 PMID:18042475

Longo, L. P., & Johnson, B. (2000). Addiction: Part I. Benzodiazepines—Side Effects, Abuse Risk and Alternatives. *American Family Physician, 61*(7), 2121–2128. https://www.aafp.org/pubs/afp/issues/2000/0401/p2121.html

Louis, V.N. & King, N. (2022). Emancipating STEM education through abolitionist teaching: A research-practice partnership to support virtual microteaching experiences. *NIH, 33*(2), 206-226.

Lourenço, R. (2001). Enteral feeding: Drug/nutrient interaction. *Clinical Nutrition (Edinburgh, Lothian)*, *20*(2), 187–193. doi:10.1054/clnu.2000.0155 PMID:11327750

Lundahl, J., Regårdh, C., Edgar, B., & Johnsson, G. (1998). The interaction effect of grapefruit juice is maximal after the first glass. *European Journal of Clinical Pharmacology*, *54*(1), 75–81. doi:10.1007002280050424 PMID:9591935

Luo, Y., Wang, C.-Z., Hesse-Fong, J., Lin, J.-G., & Yuan, C.-S. (2019). Application of Chinese Medicine in Acute and Critical Medical Conditions. *The American Journal of Chinese Medicine*, *47*(06), 1223–1235. https://doi.org/10.1142/s0192415x19500629.

Majalekar, P. P., & Shirote, P. J. (2020). Fluoroquinolones: Blessings Or Curses. *Current Drug Targets*, *21*(13), 1354–1370. doi:10.2174/1389450121666200621193355 PMID:32564750

Malhotra, S., Bailey, D. G., Paine, M. F., & Watkins, P. B. (2001). Seville orange juice-felodipine interaction: Comparison with dilute grapefruit juice and involvement of furocoumarins. *Clinical Pharmacology and Therapeutics*, *69*(1), 14–23. doi:10.1067/mcp.2001.113185 PMID:11180034

Mann, D., Gaylord, S., & Norton, S. K. (2004). *Integrating Complementary & Alternative Therapies with Conventional Care. Program on Integrative Medicine*. University of North Carolina at Chapel Hill. http://pim.med.unc.edu

McCabe, J. A., Osha, K. L., Roche, J. A., & Susser, J. A. (2013). Psychology Students' Knowledge and Use of Mnemonics. *Teaching of Psychology*, *40*(3), 183–192. doi:10.1177/0098628313487460

McLean, S.A., Caldwell, B., & Roberton, M. (2019). *Reach Out and Recover: Intentions to seek treatment in individuals using online support for eating disorders.* NIH.

Mense, E.G. (2018). The development of global higher education in a world of transformation. *NIH, 2*(3), 47.

Middle East Complementary and Alternative Medicine Market Size, Share, & Trends Analysis Report By Intervention (Traditional Alternative Medicine & Botanicals), By Application, By Distribution Channel, And Segment Forecasts, 2023 – 2030. (n.d.). https://www.grandviewresearch.com/industry-analysis/middle-east-integrative-health-complementary-alternative-medicine-market

Miller, E. L. (2002). The Penicillins: A Review And Update. *Journal of Midwifery & Women's Health*, *47*(6), 426–434. doi:10.1016/S1526-9523(02)00330-6 PMID:12484664

Miller, S. M., & Cumpston, K. L. (2014). Alpha Blockers. In *Encyclopedia of Toxicology* (pp. 154–155). Elsevier. doi:10.1016/B978-0-12-386454-3.00714-4

Minno, A., Frigerio, B., Spadarella, G., Ravani, A., Sansaro, D., Amato, M., Kitzmiller, J. P., Pepi, M., Tremoli, E., & Baldassarre, D. (2017). Old and new oral anticoagulants: Food, herbal medicines and drug interactions. *Blood Reviews*, *31*(4), 193–203 . https://doi.org/10.1016/j.blre.2017.02.001.

Miranda, L. P., Shi, L., Holder, J. R., Wright, M., Gegg, C. V., Johnson, E., Wild, K., Stenkilsson, M., Doellgast, G., Manning, B. H., & Salyers, K. (2013). Peptide antagonists of the calcitonin gene-related peptide (CGRP) receptor with improved pharmacokinetics and pharmacodynamics. *Biopolymers*, *100*(4), 422–430. doi:10.1002/bip.22270 PMID:23868210

Mohammadi, S., Asghari, G., Emami-Naini, A., Mansourian, M., & Badri, S. (2020). Herbal Supplement Use and Herb-drug Interactions among Patients with Kidney Disease. *Journal of Research in Pharmacy Practice*, *9*(2), 61–67. doi:10.4103/jrpp.JRPP_20_30 PMID:33102379

Moses, G. M., & McGuire, T. M. (2010). Drug interactions with complementary medicines. *Australian Prescriber*, *33*(6), 181. doi:10.18773/austprescr.2010.084

MQA. (2021). *Program Standards: Traditional and Complementary Medicine*. PT Online. https://www.ptonline.com/articles/how-to-get-better-mfi-results

Mueller, S. (2004). Effect of St John's wort dose and preparations on the pharmacokinetics of digoxin*1. *Clinical Pharmacology and Therapeutics*, *75*(6), 546–557. doi:10.1016/j.clpt.2004.01.014 PMID:15179409

Mujumdar, A., Dhuley, J., Deshmukh, V., Raman, P., Thorat, S., & Naik, S. (1990). Effect of piperine on pentobarbitone induced hypnosis in rats. *Indian Journal of Experimental Biology*, *28*(5), 486–487. PMID:2401524

Murre, J. M., & Dros, J. (2015). Replication and Analysis of Ebbinghaus' Forgetting Curve. *PLoS One*, *10*(7), e0120644. doi:10.1371/journal.pone.0120644 PMID:26148023

Neural academy. (2020, February 7). *CRANIAL NERVES SONG*. [Video] YouTube. https://www.youtube.com/watch?v=Omair2f46IY&t=29s

Nix, D. E., Adam, R. D., Auclair, B., Krueger, T. S., Godo, P. G., & Peloquin, C. A. (2004). Pharmacokinetics and relative bioavailability of clofazimine in relation to food, orange juice and antacid. *Tuberculosis (Edinburgh, Scotland)*, *84*(6), 365–373. doi:10.1016/j.tube.2004.04.001 PMID:15525560

Nobay, F., & Acquisto, N. M. (2014). Barbiturates. In *Encyclopedia of Toxicology* (pp. 363–367). Elsevier. doi:10.1016/B978-0-12-386454-3.00696-5

Ofer, M., Wolffram, S., Koggel, A., Spahn-Langguth, H., & Langguth, P. (2005). Modulation of drug transport by selected flavonoids: Involvement of P-gp and OCT? *European Journal of Pharmaceutical Sciences*, *25*(2-3), 263–271. doi:10.1016/j.ejps.2005.03.001 PMID:15911222

Ogata, N., Dantas, L. M., & Crowell-Davis, S. L. (2019). Selective Serotonin Reuptake Inhibitors. In *Veterinary Psychopharmacology* (pp. 103–128). Wiley. doi:10.1002/9781119226253.ch8

Owira, P. M., & Ojewole, J. A. (2010). The grapefruit: An old wine in a new glass? Metabolic and cardiovascular perspectives. *Cardiovascular Journal of Africa*, *21*(5), 280–285. PMID:20972517

Özdemir, M., Aktan, Y., Boydağ, B., Cingi, M., & Musmul, A. (1998). Interaction between grapefruit juice and diazepam in humans. *European Journal of Drug Metabolism and Pharmacokinetics*, *23*(1), 55–59. doi:10.1007/BF03189827 PMID:9625273

Page, C., Hoffman, B., Curtis, M., & Walker, M. (2006). *Integrated Pharmacology* (3rd ed.). Mosby Ltd.

Pakala, R. S., Brown, K. N., & Preuss, C. V. (2022). Cholinergic Medications. In *StatPearls*. StatPearls Publishing. https://www.ncbi.nlm.nih.gov/books/NBK538163/

Pápai, K., Budai, M., Ludányi, K., Antal, I., & Klebovich, I. (2010). In vitro food–drug interaction study: Which milk component has a decreasing effect on the bioavailability of ciprofloxacin? *Journal of Pharmaceutical and Biomedical Analysis*, *52*(1), 37–42. doi:10.1016/j.jpba.2009.12.003 PMID:20053516

Parvez, M. K., & Rishi, V. (2019). Herb-Drug Interactions and Hepatotoxicity. *Current Drug Metabolism*, *20*(4), 275–282. doi:10.2174/1389200220666190325141422 PMID:30914020

Pasi, A. K. (2013). Herb-Drug Interaction: An Overview. *International Journal of Pharmaceutical Sciences and Research*, *4*(10), 3770–3774. https://doi.org/10.13040/ijpsr.0975-8232.4(10).3770-74.

Patel, P. H., & Hashmi, M. F. (2022). Macrolides. In *StatPearls*. StatPearls Publishing. https://www.ncbi.nlm.nih.gov/books/NBK551495/

Patil, R., & Upaganlawar, A. (2020). Cholinergic Agonists. In *Advances in Neuropharmacology* (pp. 3–30). Apple Academic Press. doi:10.1201/9780429242717-2

Pattanaik, S., Hota, D., Prabhakar, S., Kharbanda, P., & Pandhi, P. (2006). Effect of piperine on the steady-state pharmacokinetics of phenytoin in patients with epilepsy. *Phytotherapy Research: An International Journal Devoted to Pharmacological and Toxicological Evaluation of Natural Product Derivatives*, *20*(8), 683–686. doi:10.1002/ptr.1937 PMID:16767797

Penzak, S. R., Acosta, E. P., Turner, M., Edwards, D. J., Hon, Y. Y., Desai, H. D., & Jann, M. W. (2002). Effect of Seville orange juice and grapefruit juice on indinavir pharmacokinetics. *Journal of Clinical Pharmacology*, *42*(10), 1165–1170. doi:10.1177/009127002237991 PMID:12362932

Platt, K., Edenharder, R., Aderhold, S., Muckel, E., & Glatt, H. (2010). Fruits and vegetables protect against the genotoxicity of heterocyclic aromatic amines activated by human xenobiotic-metabolizing enzymes expressed in immortal mammalian cells. *Mutation Research/Genetic Toxicology and Environmental Mutagenesis*, *703*(2), 90–98. doi:10.1016/j.mrgentox.2010.08.007 PMID:20713174

Polk, R. E. (1989). Drug-drug interactions with ciprofloxacin and other fluoroquinolones. *The American Journal of Medicine*, *87*(5), S76–S81. doi:10.1016/0002-9343(89)90028-4 PMID:2686430

Prior, T. I., Chue, P. S., Tibbo, P., & Baker, G. B. (1999). Drug metabolism and atypical antipsychotics. *European Neuropsychopharmacology*, *9*(4), 301–309. doi:10.1016/S0924-977X(98)00040-6 PMID:10422890

Rao, A., Shakeel, M., Trinidade, A., Rao, G., Pearce, A., & Ah-See, K-M. (2012). The Importance of Complementary and Alternative Medicine Education in Medical School. *Journal of Evidence-Based Complementary & Alternative Medicine,* 1-7. doi doi:10.1177/2156587212451597

Rodeiro, I., Donato, M., Lahoz, A., Garrido, G., Delgado, R., & Gómez-Lechón, M. (2008). Interactions of polyphenols with the P450 system: Possible implications on human therapeutics. *Mini-Reviews in Medicinal Chemistry*, *8*(2), 97–106. doi:10.2174/138955708783498131 PMID:18289092

Rodríguez-Fragoso, L., & Reyes-Esparza, J. (2013). Fruit/vegetable-drug interactions: Effects on drug metabolizing enzymes and drug transporters. *Drug Discovery*, 1-33.

Rooha, A., Anil, M. A., & Bhat, J. S. (2020). Pictures over words: A cross-sectional study reporting short term memory abilities in children. *F1000 Research*, *9*, 380. doi:10.12688/f1000research.23378.2 PMID:33520190

Roy, R., Marakkar, S., Vayalil, M. P., Shahanaz, A., Anil, A. P., Kunnathpeedikayil, S., ... Sathees, S. (2022). Drug-food Interactions in the Era of Molecular Big Data, Machine Intelligence, and Personalized Health. *Recent Advances in Food Nutrition & Agriculture*, *13*(1), 27–50. doi:10.2174/2212798412666220620104809 PMID:36173075

Russell, R. P. (1988). Side effects of calcium channel blockers. *Hypertension*, *11*(3_pt_2). doi:10.1161/01.HYP.11.3_Pt_2.II42 PMID:3280492

Sader, H. S., Rhomberg, P. R., Farrell, D. J., & Jones, R. N. (2015). Arbekacin activity against contemporary clinical bacteria isolated from patients hospitalized with pneumonia. *Antimicrobial Agents and Chemotherapy*, *59*(6), 3263–3270. doi:10.1128/AAC.04839-14 PMID:25801559

Saito, M., Hirata-Koizumi, M., Matsumoto, M., Urano, T., & Hasegawa, R. (2005). Undesirable effects of citrus juice on the pharmacokinetics of drugs: Focus on recent studies. *Drug Safety*, *28*(8), 677–694. doi:10.2165/00002018-200528080-00003 PMID:16048354

Salazar, R. (2000). How to increase your medical memory. *BMJ (Clinical Research Ed.)*, *321*, 0007245. doi:10.1136bmj.0007245

Santos, C. A., & Boullata, J. I. (2005). An approach to evaluating drug-nutrient interactions. *Pharmacotherapy: The Journal of Human Pharmacology and Drug Therapy*, *25*(12), 1789–1800. doi:10.1592/phco.2005.25.12.1789 PMID:16305298

Saravolatz, L. D., & Stein, G. E. (2015). Oritavancin: A Long-Half-Life Lipoglycopeptide. *Nephrology, Dialysis, Transplantation*, *61*(4), 627–632. https://doi.org/10.1093/cid/civ311

Sarzani, R., Salvi, F., Dessì-Fulgheri, P., & Rappelli, A. (2008). Renin–angiotensin system, natriuretic peptides, obesity, metabolic syndrome, and hypertension: An integrated view in humans. *Journal of Hypertension*, *26*(5), 831–843. doi:10.1097/HJH.0b013e3282f624a0 PMID:18398321

Scarpignato, C., Gatta, L., Zullo, A., & Blandizzi, C. (2016). Effective and safe proton pump inhibitor therapy in acid-related diseases - A position paper addressing benefits and potential harms of acid suppression. *BMC Medicine*, *14*(1), 1–35. doi:10.118612916-016-0718-z PMID:27825371

Schmid, K. L. (2021). Fluoroquinolones are a potent form of chemotherapy. *Clinical & Experimental Optometry*, *104*(3), 412–416. https://doi.org/10.1111/cxo.13102

Schmidt, L. E., & Dalhoff, K. (2002). Food-drug interactions. *Drugs*, *62*(10), 1481–1502. doi:10.2165/00003495-200262100-00005 PMID:12093316

Schmidt-Mende, K., Andersen, M., Wettermark, B., & Hasselstrom, J. (2019) Drug–disease interactions in Swedish senior primary care patients were dominated by non-steroid anti-inflammatory drugs and hypertension – a population-based registry study. *Scandinavian Journal of Primary Health Care, 38*(3), 330-339. https://doi.dtorg/10.1080/02813432.2020.1794396

Scholz, I., Liakoni, E., Hammann, F., Grafinger, K. E., Duthaler, U., Nagler, M., Krähenbühl, S., & Haschke, M. (2021). Effects of Hypericum perforatum (St John's wort) on the pharmacokinetics and pharmacodynamics of rivaroxaban in humans. *British Journal of Clinical Pharmacology*, *87*(3), 1466–1474. https://doi.org/10.1111/bcp.14553.

Schrier, R. W. (2006). Water and Sodium Retention in Edematous Disorders: Role of Vasopressin and Aldosterone. *The American Journal of Medicine*, *119*(7), S47–S53. doi:10.1016/j.amjmed.2006.05.007 PMID:16843085

Scrubssurgicalsoc. (2012, January 30). *The Twelve Cranial Nerves of Christmas*. [Video] YouTube. https://www.youtube.com/watch?v=PcQyJR4dGxc&t=80s

Scrubssurgicalsoc. (2013, September 7). *Learnthroughsong*. [Video] YouTube. https://www.youtube.com/watch?v=0lbwshg_Kj4

Secchi, A. (2022). Medication management in m inority, a sian and b lack ethnic older people in the United Kingdom: a mixed-studies systematic review. *NIH, 47*(9): p. 1322-1336.

Shah, A. U. M., Safri, S. N. A., Thevadas, R., Noordin, N. K., Rahman, A. A., Sekawi, Z., Ideris, A., & Sultan, M. T. H. (2020). COVID-19 outbreak in Malaysia: Actions taken by the Malaysian government. *International Journal of Infectious Diseases*, *97*, 108–116. doi:10.1016/j.ijid.2020.05.093 PMID:32497808

ShahrokhiM.GuptaV. (2022). Propranolol. *StatPearls*. https://www.ncbi.nlm.nih.gov/books/NBK557801/

Shaikh, S. H., Malik, F., James, H., & Abdul, H. (2009). Trends in the use of complementary and alternative medicine in Pakistan: A population-based survey. *Journal of Alternative and Complementary Medicine*, *15*(5), 545–550. doi:10.1089/acm.2008.0232 PMID:19422284

Shorvon, S. D., Andermann, F., & Guerrini, R. (2011). *The causes of epilepsy*. Cambridge University Press. doi:10.1017/CBO9780511921001

Simmons-Stern, N. R., Budson, A. E., & Ally, B. A. (2010). Music as a memory enhancer in patients with Alzheimer's disease. *Neuropsychologia*, *48*(10), 3164–3167. https://doi.org/10.1016/j.neuropsychologia.2010.04.033

Singh, A., & Zhao, K. (2017). Herb–Drug Interactions of Commonly Used Chinese Medicinal Herbs. *International Review of Neurobiology*, 197–232. doi:10.1016/bs.irn.2017.02.010

Smith, S., Newhouse, J. P., & Freeland, M. S. (2009). Income, insurance, and technology: Why does health spending outpace economic growth? *Health Affairs (Project Hope)*, *28*(5), 1276–1284. doi:10.1377/hlthaff.28.5.1276 PMID:19738242

Snyder, B. D., Polasek, T. M., & Doogue, M. P. (2012). Drug interactions: Principles and practice. *Australian Prescriber*, *35*(3), 85–88. [REMOVED HYPERLINK FIELD] doi:10.18773/austprescr.2012.037

Soliman. M. & Bilszta. J. L. (2021). Teaching complementary and alternative medicine in undergraduate medical education: a scoping review. *International Journal of Medical Education, 12,* 140-149. doi:10.5116/ijme.60e2.f3ed

Sørensen, J. M. (2002). Herb–drug, food–drug, nutrient–drug, and drug–drug interactions: Mechanisms involved and their medical implications. *Journal of Alternative and Complementary Medicine (New York, N.Y.)*, *8*(3), 293–308. doi:10.1089/10755530260127989 PMID:12165187

Spanakis, M., Patelarou, E., & Patelarou, A. (2022). Drug-Food Interactions with a Focus on Mediterranean Diet. *Applied Sciences (Basel, Switzerland)*, *12*(20), 10207. doi:10.3390/app122010207

Spiro, H. M. (1983). H2-blockers. *Journal of Clinical Gastroenterology*, *5*, 143–148. doi:10.1097/00004836-198312001-00014 PMID:6140282

Stafstrom, C. E., & Carmant, L. (2015). Seizures and Epilepsy: An Overview for Neuroscientists. *Cold Spring Harbor Perspectives in Medicine*, *5*(6), a022426–a022426. doi:10.1101/cshperspect.a022426 PMID:26033084

Steel, A. (2019). *The role and influence of traditional and scientific knowledge in naturopathic education: a qualitative study. NIH, 25*(2), p. 196-201.

Strickland, A.. (2022). What Music Reveals about Our Minds. *CNN Health*. https://www.cnn.com/2022/04/07/health/music-brain-wellness-scn

Suroowan, S., & Mahomoodally, F. (2015). Common phyto-remedies used against cardiovascular diseases and their potential to induce adverse events in cardiovascular patients. *Clinical Phytoscience*, *1*(1), 1. doi:10.118640816-015-0002-3

Suvarna, R., Pirmohamed, M., & Henderson, L. (2003). Possible interaction between warfarin and cranberry juice. *British Medical Journal*, *327*(7429), 1454. doi:10.1136/bmj.327.7429.1454 PMID:14684645

Tachjian, A., Maria, V., & Jahangir, A. (2010). Use of Herbal Products and Potential Interactions in Patients With Cardiovascular Diseases. *Journal of the American College of Cardiology*, *55*(6), 515–525. doi:10.1016/j.jacc.2009.07.074 PMID:20152556

Taddei, S., & Bruno, R. M. (2019). Calcium Channel Blockers. In *Encyclopedia of Endocrine Diseases* (pp. 689–695). Elsevier. doi:10.1016/B978-0-12-801238-3.65408-9

Taff, S. D. (2020). *Educator's guide for addressing cultural awareness, humility, and dexterity in occupational therapy curricula.* Washington University.

Tankanow, R., Tamer, H. R., Streetman, D. S., Smith, S. G., Welton, J. L., Annesley, T., Aaronson, K. D., & Bleske, B. E. (2003). Interaction Study between Digoxin and a Preparation of Hawthorn (Crataegus oxyacantha). *Journal of Clinical Pharmacology*, *43*(6), 637–642. doi:10.1177/0091270003253417 PMID:12817526

Telang, U., Ji, Y., & Morris, M. E. (2009). ABC transporters and isothiocyanates: Potential for pharmacokinetic diet–drug interactions. *Biopharmaceutics & Drug Disposition*, *30*(7), 335–344. doi:10.1002/bdd.668 PMID:19623673

Templeman, K., Robinson, A., & McKenna, L. (2015). Integrating complementary medicine literacy education into Australian medical curricula: Student-identified techniques and strategies for implementation. *Complementary Therapies in Clinical Practice, 21,* 238-246.

Thaut, M. H., Peterson, D. A., McIntosh, G. C., & Hoemberg, V. (2014). Music mnemonics aid Verbal Memory and Induce Learning - Related Brain Plasticity in Multiple Sclerosis. *Frontiers in Human Neuroscience*, *8*, 395. https://doi.org/10.3389/fnhum.2014.00395

Thomson, P., Jones, J., Evans, J. M., Stephen, L., Leslie, S. L. (2012). Factors influencing the use of complementary and alternative medicine and whether patients inform their primary care physician. *Complementary Therapies in Medicine, 20*(1–2), 45-53. https://doi.org/10.1016/j.ctim.2011.10.001

Tiec, C. L., Barrail, A., Goujard, C., & Taburet, A.-M. (2005). Clinical pharmacokinetics and summary of efficacy and tolerability of atazanavir. *Clinical Pharmacokinetics*, *44*(10), 1035–1050. doi:10.2165/00003088-200544100-00003 PMID:16176117

Tiralongo, E., & Wallis, M. (2008). Integrating Complementary and Alternative Medicine Education into the Pharmacy Curriculum. *American Journal of Pharmaceutical Education*, *72*(4), 74. doi:10.5688/aj720474 PMID:19002274

Tomasik, M.J., Helbling, L.A. & Moser, U. (2021). Educational gains of in-person vs. distance learning in primary and secondary schools: A natural experiment during the COVID-19 pandemic school closures in Switzerland. *NIH, 56*(4), 566-576.

Trescot, A. (2013). Clinical Use of Opioids. In Comprehensive Treatment of Chronic Pain by Medical, Interventional, and Integrative Approaches (pp. 99–110). Springer New York. doi:10.1007/978-1-4614-1560-2_10

Tsai, H. H., Lin, H. W., Simon Pickard, A., Tsai, H. Y., & Mahady, G. B. (2012). Evaluation of documented drug interactions and contraindications associated with herbs and dietary supplements: A systematic literature review. *International Journal of Clinical Practice*, *66*(11), 1056–1078. doi:10.1111/j.1742-1241.2012.03008.x PMID:23067030

Tyler, V. E., Brady, L. R., & Robbers, J. E. (1998). *Pharmacognosy* (9th ed.). Lea & Febiger.

Uesawa, Y., & Mohri, K. (2006). Effects of cranberry juice on nifedipine pharmacokinetics in rats. *The Journal of Pharmacy and Pharmacology, 58*(8), 1067–1072. doi:10.1211/jpp.58.8.0007 PMID:16872553

Uesawa, Y., & Mohri, K. (2008). Hesperidin in orange juice reduces the absorption of celiprolol in rats. *Biopharmaceutics & Drug Disposition, 29*(3), 185–188. doi:10.1002/bdd.603 PMID:18344215

Valenzuela, B., Rebollo, J., Pérez, T., Brugarolas, A., & Pérez-Ruixo, J. J. (2011). Effect of grapefruit juice on the pharmacokinetics of docetaxel in cancer patients: A case report. *British Journal of Clinical Pharmacology, 72*(6), 978–981. doi:10.1111/j.1365-2125.2011.04052.x PMID:21692829

Vamos, S. (2020). *Making a case for "Education for health literacy": An international perspective. MDPI, 17*(4), 1436.

Vassan, J. G. (2019). *Perceptions of Homoeopathic Practitioners Regarding Continuing Professional Development (CPD) in South Africa*. University of Johannesburg.

Verhaar, M. C., Strachan, F. E., Newby, D. E., Cruden, N. L., Koomans, H. A., Rabelink, T. J., & Webb, D. J. (1998). Endothelin-A Receptor Antagonist–Mediated Vasodilatation Is Attenuated by Inhibition of Nitric Oxide Synthesis and by Endothelin-B Receptor Blockade. *Circulation, 97*(8), 752–756. doi:10.1161/01.CIR.97.8.752 PMID:9498538

Volz, H.-P., & Gleiter, C. H. (1998). Monoamine oxidase inhibitors: A perspective on their use in the elderly. *Drugs & Aging, 13*(5), 341–355. doi:10.2165/00002512-199813050-00002 PMID:9829163

Wachtel-Galor, S. & F., I. (2011). *Herbal Medicine*. Nih.gov; CRC Press/Taylor & Francis. https://www.ncbi.nlm.nih.gov/books/NBK92773/

Walker, S. E., Shulman, K. I., Tailor, S. A., & Gardner, D. (1996). Tyramine content of previously restricted foods in monoamine oxidase inhibitor diets. *Journal of Clinical Psychopharmacology, 16*(5), 383–388. doi:10.1097/00004714-199610000-00007 PMID:8889911

Wang, H., & Leung, L. K. (2010). The carotenoid lycopene differentially regulates phase I and II enzymes in dimethylbenz [a] anthracene-induced MCF-7 cells. *Nutrition (Burbank, Los Angeles County, Calif.), 26*(11-12), 1181–1187. doi:10.1016/j.nut.2009.11.013 PMID:20400267

Wang, S. (2019). Historical Review: Opiate Addiction and Opioid Receptors. *Cell Transplantation, 28*(3), 233–238. doi:10.1177/0963689718811060 PMID:30419763

Wang, Y., & Klass, E. (2016). Grapefruit with your statin? *The American Journal of Medicine, 129*(8), e159. doi:10.1016/j.amjmed.2016.03.015 PMID:27453391

Weir, C. B., & Le, J. K. (2022). Metronidazole. In *StatPearls*. StatPearls Publishing. doi:10.1201/9781315152110

Williamson, E., Driver, S., & Baxter, K. (2009). *Stockley's herbal medicines interactions: a guide to the interactions of herbal medicines, dietary supplements, and nutraceuticals with conventional medicines*. Pharmaceutical Press.

Wong, J.T. (2022). *A learning experience design approach to online professional development for teaching science through the arts: Evaluation of teacher content knowledge, self-efficacy and STEAM perceptions,* p. 1-31. NIH.

World Health Organization. (2019). *WHO global report on traditional and complementary medicine 2019.* World Health Organization. https://apps.who.int/iris/handle/10665/312342

World Health Organization. (2021, June 11). *Cardiovascular diseases (CVDs).* WHO. https://www.who.int/news-room/fact-sheets/detail/cardio-vascular-diseases-(cvds)

Yadollah, S., Kazemipour, N., Bakhtiyari, S., & Nazifi, S. (2017). Palmitate-induced insulin resistance is attenuated by Pioglitazone and EGCG through reducing the gluconeogenic key enzymes expression in HepG2 cells. *Journal of Medicine and Life*, *10*(4), 244–249. PMID:29362600

Yu, L. X., Jiang, W., Zhang, X., Lionberger, R., Makhlouf, F., Schuirmann, D. J., Muldowney, L., Chen, M. L., Davit, B., Conner, D., & Woodcock, J. (2015). Novel bioequivalence approach for narrow therapeutic index drugs. *Clinical Pharmacology and Therapeutics*, *97*(3), 286–291. doi:10.1002/cpt.28 PMID:25669762

Zutshi, R., Singh, R., Zutshi, U., Johri, R., & Atal, C. (1985). Influence of piperine on rifampicin blood levels in patients of pulmonary tuberculosis. *The Journal of the Association of Physicians of India*, *33*(3), 223–224. PMID:4044481

About the Contributors

Muhammad Shahzad Aslam is a young high-performing professional with more than ten years of experience in higher education. He is currently working as Assistant Professor in the School of Traditional Chinese Medicine, Xiamen University Malaysia. He completed his PhD from Universiti Malaysia Perlis, Malaysia, under a scholarship awarded by the Government of Malaysia under the Ministry of Higher Education Malaysia categorized as Malaysian International Scholarship. He had completed M.Phil in Pharmaceutical Chemistry from Bahauddin Zakariya University, Multan, Pakistan. He has graduated as a Doctor of Pharmacy (Pharm-D) from Baqai Medical University, Karachi, Pakistan. He has been working with a multidisciplinary attitude in digital health, mental health, psychopharmacology, public health, natural product chemistry, green chemistry, novel extraction prototype, extraction, fractionation and isolation of bioactive compounds, stabilities studies of pharmaceuticals, standardization of herbal product, pre-clinical trials, and health informatics. The researcher currently working to identify new biomolecules in chronic pain and rare neurological disorders. Currently, he has an h index fourteen (14) and i10 index seventeen (17). During his small scientific carrier, the researcher had published more than 85 articles in international peer-review journals and had collaborated with different universities such as the Centro Escolar University, Malaysian Agricultural Research and Development Institute (MARDI), University of Tabuk, Saudi Arabia, Universiti Utara Malaysia, Sintok, Malaysia, Department of Pharmacology & Toxicology, University of Veterinary and Animal Sciences, Lahore, Pakistan, Girijananda Chowdhury Institute of Pharmaceutical Science, Guwahati, India, University of Lahore, Pharmaceutical Academy, Russia. He was nominated as the top 1% reviewer in clinical medicine and cross-discipline in 2019. He has reviewed more than 462+ articles and had handle 274+ articles as an academic editor. He was consistent top reviewer in 2018 and 2017. He is currently serving as an academic editor in prestigeous journal (i.e., PLOS, Medicine, Frontiers in Clinical Diabetes and Healthcare).

* * *

Mohammad Ayaz Ahmad completed Ph.D. in Experimental High Energy Physics in 2010 and M. Phil. (Physics) in 2005 from the Physics Department, Aligarh Muslim University, Aligarh, India. I worked as a Guest Lecturer for B. Sc. Laboratory Classes in the same Department, Aligarh Muslim University, Aligarh w.e.f. 10th Oct. 2002 to 10th Oct. 2008 and also as a Lecturer at Senior Secondary College (Boy's) of Aligarh Muslim University, Aligarh w.e.f. 11th Oct. 2008 to 15th Dec. 2010. I worked as an Assistant Professor at University of Tabuk, D.O.F. Physics from 16th Dec. 2010 to 28th December, 2021. And recently, I started working as a Professor at University of Guyana, Georgetown, South America D.O.F. Physics w.e.f. 1st September 2022.

Yun Jin Kim has a Ph.D. degree from Second medical college, Nanjing University of Traditional Chinese Medicine, Nanjing, Jiangsu Province, China in 2009. His Ph.D. project and thesis supported by the National Natural Science Foundation of China (NSFC, Grant No.: 90209027/H2718). The biomedical researcher has done by the Department of Physics, Seoul National University, Seoul, Korea. His research project supported by the Ministry of Science and Technology, Korea & Cavendish-KAIST Cooperative Research Program. More than 10 years of TCM clinical experience and teaching in the higher education institutions in Malaysia. Currently, an Associate professor of the School of Traditional Chinese Medicine at Xiamen University Malaysia, Selangor, Malaysia. He has been listed among the World's Top 2% Scientist 2021 by Stanford University (H-Index: 58). Ongoing Scientific Activities include (1) Clinical assessment of Complementary medicine; (2) Complementary medicine educational environment for clinical practice; (3) Epidemiology & Public health, i.e. neurologic disorders / mental health; (4) Longevity; (5) Integrative medicine clinical service for Neurology; (6) Ongoing clinical trial topics are Acupuncture for Anxiety in Parkinson's disease (NCT04729010) and Efficacy of Moxibustion in Diabetes Peripheral Neuropathy (NCT04894461).

Qian Linchao graduated from Fujian University of Traditional Chinese Medicine in 1985. He is now a professor of Traditional Chinese Medicine at Xiamen University Malaysia, the vice dean of Xiamen University, School of Medicine and the dean of School of traditional Chinese Medicine, Xiamen University Malaysia. He has been engaged in clinical medicine and teaching of traditional Chinese Medicine for more than 30 years. He is engaging with basic and clinical research on spleen and stomach and cardiovascular disease and has published more than 50 research papers.

Syed Khalid Mustafa completed Ph.D. in Organic Chemistry in 2004 from the Chemistry Department, Patna University, India, Presently, working in Department of Chemistry, Faculty of Science, University of Tabuk, Saudi Arabia since past several years. He has published more than 25 research articles in various National and International Journals.

Index

A

Adverse Drug Reactions 25, 33, 39, 134
Allied Health 118
Aloe Vera 136
Aspirin 11, 97, 100, 130, 149

B

Bioaccumulation 153
Bioengineering 40
Biotherapeutics 53

C

Chan Su 130
Clinical Western Medicine 38, 40
Complementary Medicine 18-20, 36, 66, 70, 72, 116, 124, 128, 137-138
Cranial Nerves Song 108-109, 114

D

Dan Shen 130
Dietary Substances 22, 24, 28-29
Digoxin 11, 14, 25, 30, 130, 133-135, 137-140
Drug Interactions 1, 3-13, 16-19, 29-31, 33, 36, 39, 134, 140, 149
Drug-Food Interactions 1, 6, 14, 36
Drug-Herb Interactions 13, 23, 130, 133
Drugs 1, 4-19, 21-29, 32, 36-37, 39, 42-46, 66-71, 73-74, 76, 80, 84-85, 90, 93-94, 100-101, 104, 110, 112, 130-137, 139-140, 142, 148, 151

E

Educating 18, 66, 118-119, 121, 125

F

Food Supplements 21-22, 29

G

Garlic 14
Ginseng 17, 135

H

Heavy Metal Contaminations 150

I

Interactions 1, 3-19, 22-25, 27-33, 35-36, 39, 122-123, 125, 130-131, 133-145, 147-149, 182

M

Medical Education 18, 20, 74, 104, 118, 128
Medical Rhymes 106, 114
Milk and Dairy Products 151-153, 167, 181
Mnemonics 45, 66-67, 73-74, 99, 102, 104, 106, 110-111, 114-115
Music 45, 104-106, 108-111, 113-115

P

Papaya Leaf 62

Pharmacokinetic Interactions 138
Pharmacological Evidence 130, 141
Pharmacology 1, 3-4, 19, 29-47, 49-52, 64, 66, 70-71, 74, 100-101, 104, 110-111, 113-114, 116, 118, 131, 137-140, 147-149
Pharmacy 17, 19-20, 30-31, 36, 39, 46, 61, 64, 123, 125-127, 139

S

Songs 73-74, 105-106, 109-113
Squalene 54-65
Students 1, 3-4, 18, 38-47, 53, 66-67, 73-99, 102, 104-106, 108-111, 113, 116-123, 125-128

T

Technology 2, 19, 54, 63-64, 116-117, 121-123, 128, 150, 156
Traditional Chinese Medicine 38-41, 43, 46, 53, 58, 66-67, 73-74, 121, 131, 141-142, 149

U

Undergraduate 20, 38-43, 45-47, 49, 52, 73-74, 129

W

Warfarin 23, 26, 36
Wound 54-60, 62-64

www.ingramcontent.com/pod-product-compliance
Lightning Source LLC
LaVergne TN
LVHW081519300926
849161LV00006B/1227
* 9 7 8 1 6 6 8 4 7 8 2 8 8 *